VAGUS NERVE

A guide to stimulate and activate your vague nerve through self-help exercises to alleviate anxiety

By

RYKER PLACID

reparation, damage, or financial misfortune is incurred either directly or by implication because of the data contained in this.

Particular creators claim all copyrights not held by the distributor.

The data in this is offered for educational purposes exclusively and is all-inclusive as so. The introduction of the data is without a contract or any sort of assurance confirmation.

The trademarks that are utilized are with no assent, and the distribution of the trademark is without consent or support by the trademark proprietor. All trademarks and brands inside this book are for explaining purposes just and are simply possessed by the proprietors, not partnered with this record.

TABLE OF CONTENTS

INTRODUCTION

Simply put, the vagus nerve is the supreme commander of your inner nerve center and regulates all your major organs. This is the longest ever cranial that starts behind the ears in the brain and interacts with all major bodies. This sends fibers, and actually directs the inner core of your nerve, to all your visceral organs, sending nerve impulses to every organ in your body. The term vagus means, basically, "hiking" because it stretches from the brain to the reproductive organs all over the body. The vagus nerve, except the surrender and thyroid glans, is important in connection with the mental body as it passes all major organs.

For each organ, it is in contact; this is an essential nerve. It helps prevent anxiety and depression in the brain. The reason for our response to each other is closely connected to the vaguely attached nervous system that adapts our ore to speak and coordinates eye contact and gestures. This nerve can also affect the correct release of hormones in the body to maintain a healthy mind and body system.

The vagus nerve increases the acidity of the stomach and digestive juice production to promote digestion in the stomach. It can also help you absorb vitamin B12 when activated. If it does not work properly, you can then expect serious intestinal problems like Colitis, IBS, and Re-flux, only to name a few. Re-flux problems are caused by a vagus nerve problem because the esophagus is also regulated. It is the insufficient esophagus reflection that triggers conditions such as Gerd and Re-flux.

The vagus nerve also helps to prevent heart rate and blood pressure. In the liver and pancreas, the balance of blood glucose, avoiding diabetes, is regulated by this nerve. The vagus nerve helps to release bile when it travels through the gallbladder, which allows the body to absorb toxins and split fat. In the bladder, it is this nerve that facilitates improved kidney function, increases blood flow, and thus improves our body's filtration. When the vagus nerve is reached through activation, inflammation in all target organs will be minimized. That nerve even has the ability to control female fertility and orgasms. An inactive or blocked vagus nerve may cause havoc through the mind and body.

Now that we know that the vagus nerve is connected to all the main organs and their proper functioning, we easily conclude that any mental or body or spirit disability, sickness, or disease can be reversed or even cured by triggering and improving the vagus nerve. You can also have positive effects on conditions like anxiety, heart disease, depression and migraine, fibromyalgia, alcohol addiction, digestion, gut problems, memory problems, mood disorders, MS, and even cancer.

Vagus nerves can be activated by many recorded forms, such as singing or chanting, music, yoga, meditation, respiratory exercises, general exercise, and just to name a couple. Singing and laughing activate the muscles behind the mouth, stimulating the nerve. Mild exercise and rehabilitation generally increase intestinal fluids, which activate the vagus nerve. Regimented yoga may also improve nerve activation due to movement, but meditation and OM-ing can also enhance vagus nerve function. All this activates the vagus nerve and has one thing in common: tone! Tone!!

Physicians are found to help vibrate the body into a state of health globally and move illness and illnesses such as anxiety, PTSD, migraines, depression, memory problems, chronic pain, sleep problems, and cancer. Dr. Gaynor, director of ontology at the Strang Cornell Cancer Prevention Center in New York and author of Sounds of Healing, said: "You can truly see the disease as a form of disharmony. "We know that the music and the sound have profound effects on the immune system that obviously has much to do with cancer." A study was also conducted in April 2016 involving Alzheimer's patients. Researchers at the University of Toronto, the Wilfrid Laurier University and Hospitals Baycrest Center conducted the study in various phases of the disease and subjected these patients to a 40-hertz sound simulation. With awareness, comprehension, and alertness, they noted "promising" outcomes. "Sections in the brain seem to be at the same contact level, and the frequency is about 40 Hz. So, when you have the malfunction-if you have too little of it-both parts of the brain that want to communicate, like the Thalamus and hippocampus, the short-lasting remembering for long-lasting memory, you can't do that. Tomatis claimed to have handled a wide range of diseases effectively by the sound because they were all linked to inner ear issues. Just a few of the conditions he has successfully treated include stuttering, depression, Adhd, concentration problems, and coordination disorders.

Another study indicates that the Tomatis approach benefits children with ADD. "These studies have shown substantial improvements in Tomatis's processing speed, phonologic understanding, and phonemic decoding efficacy compared with non-Tomatis: the sound group quickly became the most inflamed about alternative healthcare providers. Sound is an outstanding application of traditional medicine to activate the vagus nerve and enhance the body's health and vitality. Do that through Crystal Chakra Singing Bowls and Sound Healing. Clear quartz is called the' Master Healer,' as it can enhance, transform, and relay energy. The impacts in these quartz crystal bowls are intensive on organs, tissues, cells, and on the circulatory, endocrine, and metabolic systems. The crystal pulse is heard by the ear and feels within the body, stimulates the nerve in all the centers of the chakra, which induces harmony and rejuvenation of skin, body and mind.

HISTORICAL NOTE AND TERMINOLOGY

In the mid-twentieth century, electrical stimulation of the vagus nerve for epilepsy arose from findings that such stimulation could cause EEG improvements, but the first clinical use of electrical vagus nerve stimulation for epileptics was in the late nineteenth century. In the 1880s, a transcutaneous electrical stimulus for the prophylactic and abortive treatment of seizures was created to be applied over the carotid artery. The basis of this treatment was that bilateral carotid artery compression aborted seizures at the end of the 18th century. Such treatments were supported by the belief that seizures were caused by excessive brain blood flow. These therapies were discontinued the subsequent development of pharmacologic treatments for epilepsy.

Stimulation of the vagus nerve is currently used and dates back to 1952, where interictal spikes in a strychnine model of feline epilepsy can be prevented. Vagus nerve boost interest as a modern therapy for epilepsy was confirmed 30 years later, evidenced by the antiepileptic effect of vagus nerve stimulation that produces electrical stimuli in canine epilepsy models Strychnine and Pentylenetetrazol. More animal studies in rats verified this effect, encouraged the quest for optimal stimulus parameters, and launched the human experiments.

The first human stimulator implantation started clinical therapy in 1988 and continued on with major studies and randomized controlled trials for the next 8 years. For use in clinical trials and later clinical practice, a number of similar stimulators (neurocybernetic prostheses) have been developed. Such machines are the only means available to activate the therapeutic vagus nerve. It was approved in the United States for focal epilepsy treatment in 1997 and for treatment for therapeutic resistant depression in 2005. Since 2018, the neurocybernetic prosthesis has been implanted and used in 70 countries in over 100,000 people worldwide.

The first VNS system was installed in the USA in 1988. Regulatory authorization as an alternative treatment to minimize the seizure frequency was given in Europe in 1994 and in the USA in 1997. Australia's first implant was in 1994, and the Therapeutic Goods Administration (Australia) gave regulatory approval in April 2000. Globally, more than 20,000 people have implanted a VNS, of which 5,500 are under the age of 18. A total of 146 people in Australia have had a VNS implant since 1994, 66 of whom are girls. The unit was

replaced in 13 adults and 5 children after the end of the
life of the battery.

THE VAGUS NERVE: YOUR BODY'S COMMUNICATION SUPERHIGHWAY

The vagus nerve acts as the superpath of the body, carries information between the brain and the inner organs, and controls the body.'

The great nerve emerges from the brain and branches in several directions to the neck and the chest, where it brings sensory information from the skin of the ear and regulates muscles you use to swallow and move, and affects the immune system.

According to the Encyclopedia Britannica, the vagus is the 10th of 12 cranial nerves originating from the brain. Although the vagus nerve is called solitary, in fact, it has two nerves from the right and left of the oblong medulla portion of your brain truncation. The nerve is known for running according to Merriam-Webster because the vagus is the largest and the wildest cranial nerve.

The vagus nerve, roaming and ramifying across the body, represents the main influence of the sympathetic division of the nervous system: the rest and digestion of the sympathetic nervous system's combat / flight response. The unclear nerve sends signals that increase the appetite and regulate the heart and breathing rate when the body is not nervous. During stress cycles, management switches to the mechanism of compassion with the opposite effect.

The vagus nerve also brings sensory signals back into the brain from the internal organs, allowing the brain to track the activities of the organ.

The brain-good axis Large parts of the vagus nerve spread to the digestive system. According to the textbook ' Nerves and nerve injury Volume 1' (Academic Press, 2015), about 10% to 20% of vagus nerve cells attached to a digestive system transmit control commands from the brain to guide muscles that pass food through the intestines. The muscles are then regulated by a different nervous system inside the walls of the digestive system.

The other 80% to 90% of the neurons bring sensory information from the intestines and stomach to the brain. It is called a brain-good axis and holds the brain up-to-date on the status of the contraction of muscles, the speed of food passage through the stomach, and the feelings of starvation and satiety. Studying the vagus nerve with the digestive system was found to improve nerve stimulation syndrome in 2017 published in the Journal of Internal Medicine. In the Journal of Internal Medicine

Over recent decades, several scientists have found that there is a different parallel to that brain-good axis—the bacteria residing inside the intestines. According to a review published in 2014 in Advances in Experimental Medicine and Biology, this microbiota interacts with the brain through the vagus nerve, influencing not only food intake but mood and inflammation. Much of the current research includes studies of mice and rats instead of humans. However, the findings are compelling and demonstrate that microbiome changes can cause brain changes.

Vagus nerve stimulation, as a medical intervention Vagus nerve stimulation, has worked in the treatment of epilepsy cases not reacting to medications. Surgeons put an electrode into the neck, with the battery implanted under the collarbone, around the right branch of the vagus nerve. According to the Epilepsy Foundation, the electrode provides regular nerve stimulation that reduces or rarely prevents excessive brain activity that causes seizures. A vagus nerve stimulator has been approved by Europe that needs no operational implantation.

Studies have also shown that vagus nerve stimulation can be successful without medications in the treatment of psychiatric conditions. Regarding treatment-resistant stress and cluster headaches, the FDA has approved Vagus nerve stimulation. The results on behavioral resistant anxiety disorders such as obsessive-compulsive disorder, panic disorder, and post-traumatic stress disorder were reported in a 2008 brain stimulation test.

Researchers have studied the role of the Vagus Nerve in chronic inflammatory disorders, such as sepsis, lungs, Rheumatoid Arthritis (RA), and diabetes, in a new report in the Journal of Inflammation Research. Due to its impact on the immune system, the vagus nerve can cause nerve damage to autoimmune and other disorders.

Damage to the vagus' nerve, Scientists have long known that chronic diseases such as alcohol and diabetes can affect nerves, including the vagus. Neuropathy can occur in many nerves in persons with insulin-dependent diabetes. If the vagus nerve is weakened, it may cause nausea, blossoming, diarrheas, and gastroparesis. Unfortunately, diabetic neuropathy can't be reversed.

The vagus nerve is partly responsible for someone who is mildly cold, stands long, or is shocked by something uncomfortable, like brain vision. Internal detachment opens the internal blood vessels, and the vagus' nerve overreacts, leading to a quick and fast weakening of the heart rate. Blowing on the legs and the weight decreases. Without adequate blood flow to the brain, the person loses consciousness temporarily. Any medicines are required for a vasovagal syncope unless a person faints periodically.

AXIS IN PSYCHIATRIC AND INFLAMMATORY DISORDERS VAGUS NERVE AS BRAIN-GUT

The vagus is a major component of the nervous system, controlling various vital functions of the body, including mood control, immune response, metabolism, and cardiovascular performance. It transmits information about the internal organ status by afferent fibers to the brain and forms a bond between the brain and the GIV. they deal with certain unclear nervous systems in the treatment of neurological and gastrointestinal conditions. Apparently. Preliminary evidence of effective possible treatment for refractive regeneration, post-traumatic stress disorder, and vagus nerve sensational inflammatory bowel disease.

Vagus nerve stimulation improves the tone of the vagus and lowers the production of cytokine. Both of these are important resistance mechanisms. Vagal fiber activation affects the monoaminergic mechanisms in the brain, which play a significant role in severe psychiatric conditions like depression and anxiety. In specific, it is the initial proof of positive mood and anxiety effects, partially by vagus nerve activity, on intestinal bacteria. Meditations and Yoga can influence the vagal tone, which can lead to the ability to manage stress response and respiration and minimize the symptoms of mood and anxiety.

A complex system is used to link the brain with the gastrointestinal tract (the' true axis'), bidirectional (for example, prevertebral ganglia), as well as to sympathizes with endocrine and digestive interactions and with the effect of gut microbiota in gastrointestinal homeostasis. There are more than 30 neurotransmitters and more neurons in the ENS than the brain. Blood-brain membranes (e.g., ghrelin) cross hormones and peptides that trigger ENS into the bloodstream and can act with the vaginal nerve to control, for example, digestion and appetite. The diagnosis of pathological and gastrointestinal disorders, for example, inflammatory bowel disease (IBD), depression, and PTSD become more and more important in the relationship between brain and good.

The intestine is an important immune system control center, and the slight neuron has immunomodulatory characteristics. The nerve plays an important role in your intestine, brain, and inflammation as well. New therapy methods such as VNS and meditation strategies are available for stimulating the brain-good axis. Such treatments were proven to be effective in other highly inflammable situations and not only in mood and anxiety disorders. In reality, well-directed pulmonary hypnotherapy has proved to be both irritable bowel syndrome and IBD. A strong link between dietetic and mental, physiological, and inflammatory disorders is also the vagus nerve.

Basic Vagus Nerve Anatomy

The vagus nerve has a wide range of signals, extending from the digestive system and the liver to the cortex. It is the tenth cranial nerve to pass through the neck and thorax from its origins through the brainstem to the abdomen. It is also referred to by its long way through the human body as the "wandering nerve."

In the groove between the olive and the brain peduncle, a vagal nerve is removed from the medulla oblongata. The brain occupies the center part of the foramen. The vagal nerve in the neck supplies a vacuum necessary to swallow and vocalize the majority of the pharynx and larynx muscles. In the thorax, the heart gets the main part of sympathy that induces heart rate reduction. The vagus nerve of the bowel regulates the activity and secretion of the glutinous muscle. Efferent vagal neurons produce the muscular and molecular structures of the intestines through the vagus motor core in vagus nerve medulla and inert to the lamina propria as well as external muscular structures.

The celiac branch supplies the intestine with the distal colon component from the proximal duodenum. The vagal gastrointestinal afferents include mucosal mechanoreceptors, chimney receptors, and oesophageal, uterine, and proximate small intestinal tightening receptors. In node ganglia, receptive cell bodies have information about nuclear tract solitaries (NTS). In several CNS areas, the NTS guided sensory vagal feedback such as the Locus coeruleus (LC) area, the Rostral Medulla, the Thalamus area, and the Amygdala region.

The vagus nerve controls the inner working of the brain, such as digestion, heart rate, breathing rate, movement of the vasomotor, and certain reflections, such as cough, sneezing, chewing, and vomiting. The synaptic junction between the neurons, the nerve fibers, and the smooth muscles is formed by acetylcholine (ACh). ACh connects with the muscle contractions of the nicotine, muscarin, and sympathetic nervous system.

Animal studies demonstrated an outstanding performance of nerve vagus regeneration. Subdiaphragmatic vagotomy, for example, facilitated the transient elimination and regeneration in the NTS of central vagus contaminants and synaptic plasticity. In comparison, the efferent reinnervation of the gastrointestinal tract is not yet recovered after 45 weeks, 18 weeks after vaginal diaphragm recuperation can be achieved.

VAGUS NERVE FUNCTIONS

The role of Vagus in autonomous nervous system functions

The parasympathetic nervous system constitutes one of the three branches of the autonomic nervous system between the sympathetic nervous system and the enteric nervous system (ENS).

The definition is primarily anatomical of nervous sympathy and part sympathy systems. The primary connection with the nervous system is the vagus nerve. The nervous oculomotor, the nerve facial, and the nervous glossopharyngeal are three parasympathetic cranial nerves.

The vagus nerve's main function is to remind the brain of the internal organs, such as the intestines, kidneys, heart, and lungs. This means that the inner organs provide the brain with vital sensory information. The intestine is the highest surface towards the outside world and, therefore, a sensory organ of particular importance.

The vagus has been traditionally studied as an efferent nerve and a sympathetic nervous system antagonist. The vagus nerve and sympathetic efferents through the splanchnic nerves are normal to many organs. The parasympathetic nervous system, together with the sympathetic nervous systems, controls vegetative processes by behaving in opposition. Parasympathetic innervation causes blood vessels and bronchioles to widen and salivary glands to intensify. On the opposite, sympathetic innervation leads to blood vessels constricting, bronchial dilating, heart rate rises, and intestinal and urinary sphincter limits. Parasympathetic nervous system activation increases bowel motility and glandular seclusion in the gastrointestinal system. By comparison, sympathetic action decreases bowel function and reduces blood supply to the gut, which causes higher blood flow to the heart and muscles as people face existential stress.

The ENS emerges from predominantly vagal neural crest cells, comprising of a nerve plexus located in the intestinal wall, spreading from the esophagus to the anus across the whole gastrointestinal tract. The human ENS is thought to contain about 100-500 million neurons. This is the biggest cell build-up in the human body. As the ENS is the shape, function, and chemical coding identical to the brain, it was defined as a "second brain" or a "brain in the gut." It consists of two ganglionated plexuses, the plexus submucous, which regulates the gastrointestinal blood flow and controls the epithelial cell and the secretion and the myenteric plexus.

ENS functions as an intestinal membrane and controls main enteric processes such as immune response, recognition of nutrients, motility, microvascular drainage and blood, Ion, and bioactive peptide epithelial secretion. There is obviously "contact" between the vagal nerve and the ENS, and cholinergic stimulation via the nicotine receptors is the key transmitter. The link between ENS and the vagal nerve in the CNS leads to a two-way flow of data. The ENS, on the other hand, also operates entirely independently of the vaguely-regulated intestinal system because it includes full reflex channels, including sensory neurons and motor neurons. We control muscle activity and motility, fluid flow, mucous membrane flow and the work of the mucous barrier. In the cells of the adaptive and innate immune systems, ENS neurons are also in close contact and controlling their activities and actions. ENS aging and cell death are associated with symptoms like constipation, incontinence and evacuation conditions. Valve-threatening depletion of

ENS in the small and large intestines (Hirschsprung's disease; pseudo-obstruction of the gut).

The connection between the CNS and the ENS, also called the brain-gout axis, helps the brain to connect with the gastrointestinal system. It regulates physiologic homeostasis in the brain's emotional and cognitive regions, including immunization, to the external intestinal functions. The axis for neurogood consists of the spinal cord, the brain, the adaptive nervous system, and HPA. These gray efferents relay signals from the brain to the intestine by means of powerful fibers that account for 10-20% of all fibers, while from the intestine to the spines 80-90% of all fibers.

The vagal afferent pathways include the activation / regulation of the HPA axis that regulates the organism's adaptive responses to stressors of any kind. In addition to elevated systemic proinflammatory cytokines, environmental stress stimulates the HPA axis by removing the CRF from the hypothalamus. Freedom of CRF stimulates the ACTH (adrenocorticotropic hormone) secretion from the pituitary disease. Such activation contributes in effect to the release of cortisol from the surreal glands. Cortisol is an essential stress hormone, affecting a wide number of human organs, including the brain, teeth, muscles, and body fat.

The brain controls all communication lines, including the immune cells, epithelial, enteral neurons, smooth muscles, Cajal cells, or enterocollate cells, between the neural (vagus) and hormonal (HPA) cells for the productive activity of the intestinal effector. The intestinal microbiota, on the other hand, affects these cells. The gut microbiota is essential for the brain-gout axis and directly affects neuroendocrine and metabolizing processes and interacts with intestinal cells and ENS locally. Emerging data support the microbiota's role in anxiety and depression. Work on germ-free animals has shown that microbiota causes stress reactivity and anxiety-like actions and controls the HPA function. In fact, these individuals are less nervous, with higher ACTH and cortisol levels and rising stress response.

For the intake of food, vagal afferents that communicate with the gastrointestinal tube provide a fast and distinct account of both digestible food and circulating and stored fuels. In conjunction with hormonal pathways, vagal efferents co-determine the nutrient absorption, accumulation, and mobilization rate. Histological, as well as electrophysiological evidence, shows a number of chemical and mechanosensitive receptors mediated by visceral afferent ends of the intestinal vagus nerve. Such receptors are the products of intestinal hormones and control peptides released from the enteroendocrine gastrointestinal system by nutrient distension and neuronal signals. We affect food intake management and the regulation of satiety, gastric emptying, and energy balance by sending signals from the upper intestines to the nucleus of the brain's solitary tract. The bulk of these hormones, such as peptide cholecystokinin (CCK), ghrelin, and leptin, are immune to the nutrient in the gut and help regulate short-term appetite and satiety feelings.

Cholecystokinin regulates gastrointestinal functions, including gastric emptying and food intake inhibition, by activating CCK-1 receptors in vagal afferent intestinal fibers. CCK is also essential for pancreatic fluid separation and gastric acid development, gallbladder contraction, gastric emptying decrease, and digestion facilitation. Saturated fat, long-chain fatty acids, amino acids, and low protein synthesis peptides are the sources of the CCK escape from the small intestines. There are several biologically active types of CCK identified by their number of amino acids, i.e., CCK-5, CCK-8,CCK-22,CCK-33. CCK-8 often prevails in neurons, while the endocrine gut cells include a combination of smaller and larger CCK peptides, often mainly CCK-33 or CCK-22.

Among rodents, both long-and short-chain food fatty acids cause, therefore, jejunal vaginal, afferent nerve fibers. Short-chain fatty acids, for example, butyric acid, directly affect vagal afferent terminals, while long-chain fatty acids cause CCK-dependant vagal afferents. The exogenous administration of CCK tends to suppress the endogenous secretion of CCK. In enteric vagus nerves, pre-frontal cortexes, thalamus, hypothalamus, basal ganglia, and dorsal hindbrain, CCK is also active as a neurotransmitter. It activates vagal afferent ends in the NTS directly by increasing the release of calcium. There is also evidence to show that CCK may stimulate neurons in the hindbrain and intestinal myenteric (a plexus that offers motor internalization to both levels of the gut's muscular layer), rats and CCK-induced Fos (a form of proto-oncogenic) expression in the brain is attenuated by vagotomy or capsaïcin therapy. There is also significant evidence that higher CCK levels induce anxiety feelings. CCK is therefore used in humans and animals as a test tool for modeling anxiety disorders.

Ghrelin is another hormone released from the belly, which plays a key role in promoting the intake of food by inhibiting vagal afferent firing. The circulating level of ghrelin is increased by fasting and decrease after a meal. Central or peripheral administration of acylated ghrelin to rats increases acute food intake, and the release of growth hormones and chronic administration leads to increased weight. Ghrelin's function in the feeding of a particular afferent neurotoxin, vagotomy or procedure, is eliminated or attenuated. In humans, infusion or subcutaneous injection increases both the feeling of starvation and the dietary intake because ghrelin suppresses the release of insulin. It is, therefore, not shocking that obesity and insulin resistance are affected by secretion.

In the vagus nerve, leptin receptors were also identified. Rotent studies show specifically that leptin and CCK work synergistically to cause short-term food intake reduction and long-term body weight loss. The epithelial cells that respond both to ghrelin and leptin are located close to the vagal mucosal endings and modulate the activity of vagal addictions to regulate intakes of food together. Amid rapid and dietary obesity in mouse, leptin is losing its potential impact on vagal mucosal afferents.

The gastrointestinal tract is the central interface between food and the human body and, through specific G-protein-coupling taste receptors, can detect essential tastes in the same way as the voice. Different taste qualities cause various gastric peptides to be released. Bitter taste receptors can be seen as possible hunger elimination targets by facilitating the release of CCK. Actually, stimulation of bitter flavor receptors triggers ghrelin release and thus the vagus nerve.

Nerve Vagus as Intestinal Immune Homeostasis Modulator

The gastrointestinal tract has a constant risk of diet and bacteria antigens, as well as symbiotic intestinal microbiota. Vaginal fibers connect the chronic neuroendocrine-immune axis with the intestinal immune system and make vagus a key component. It's completely intractable. This axis results in neuronal, behavioral, and endocrine synchronized responses that are crucial in the first line of inflammatory protection. For example, activated macrophages, dendritic cells, and other mucosal cells are formed by tumor necrosis factor-alpha (T NF-α) in response to pathogenic agents and other adverse factors. TNF-α, together with prostaglandins and interferons, is an important mediator for local and systemic inflammation. The source of cardinal clinical inflammation, including burning, swelling, discomfort, and redness, also improves. Counter-regulatory mechanisms, such as immunological cells and anti-inflammatory cytokines, typically inhibit acute inflammatory responses and prohibit inflammatory mediators from spreading into the bloodstream. In fact, a "hard-wired" link occurs between the nervous system and the immune system as an anti-inflammatory mechanism. The complex of the dorsal vagus, composed of the sensory nuclei, postrema and dorsal motor nucleus of the vagus, responds to an increase in TNF-α circulating levels by modifying muscle function in the vagus nerve.

Three specific mechanisms mediate the anti-inflammatory ability of the vagus nerve. The first direction is the above mentioned HPA axis. The second way is the splenic sympathetic antiinflammatory pathway through which the vagus nerve activates the splenic nerve. At the distal end of the splenic nerve, norepinephrine (NE) (noradrenaline) is introduced into the β2 adrenergic receptor of splenic lymphocytes that produce ACh. Finally, ACh inhibits TNF-α release via α-7-nicotinic ACh receptors by spleen macrophages. The last route, called CAIP, is via vagal efferent fibers that synapse into enteric neurons and, in turn, release ACh at the synaptic junction with macrophages. To order to block the TNF-α, ACh binds to α-7-nicotinic ACh receptors of these macrophages. The CAIP, compared to the HPA axis, provides a certain number of unique features such as an instant module entrance into the inflammatory area with a high neural conductance score. The CAIP plays an important role in intestinal immune response and homeostasis and is particularly interested in developing new treatments of inflammatory disorders associated with the intestinal immune system.

Inflammatory reflexes are the main components of the above mentioned inflammatory sensing or inflammatory suppressing processes. Innate cytokine-releasing immune cells are activated by the development of pathogens. It activates the sensory fibers that climb to the nucleus tractus solitarius in the vagus nerve. Cutting down efferent signals in the vagus nerve by the macrophage nicotine receptor and the CAIP inhibits the production of peripheral cytokines. Experimental CAIP activation increases the TNF α development of the liver, spleen, and heart by direct electrical stimulation of the efferent vagus nerve and delays the Serum TNF α concentrations.

Stimulation of the vagus nerve

Vagus nerve stimulation is a routine medical procedure for seizures and other neurological conditions. VNS tests are not only clinically but also scientifically insightful about the health and disease function of the vagus nerve.

Method and tool

Vagus nerve stimulation occurs through the use of electrical impulses in the vagus nerve. The activation of the vagus nerve can be achieved in two ways: overt surgical stimulation, usually the most common use, and an indirect non-invasive transcutaneous stimulation. Invasive VNS (iVNS) requires operative implantation in the left thoracic region of a small pulse generator. The electrodes are attached to the vagus nerve of the left cervix and connected by a plumb to the pulse generator tunneled under the skin. The motor sends electrical pulses to the brain through the vagus nerve. Such electrical pulses are expected to have antiepileptic, antidepressant, and anti-inflammatory effects by modifying nerve cell excitability. Contrary to iVNS, transcutaneous VNS (tVNS) enables a non-invasive vagus nerve stimulation without surgery.

The stimulator is usually connected to the auricular concha via an ear clip, which delivers electrical impulses on the subcutaneous path of the vagus nerve's afferent auricular division. A pilot study investigating the use of VNS in 60 patients with treatment-resistant depression has shown a substantial therapeutic change and good tolerability in 30-37% of patients. Five years later, the US allowed the activation of the vagus nerve to relieve refractory depression. Administration of Food and Drugs (FDA). Several observational studies have since shown the safety and efficacy of VNS in depression, as can be seen below. In fact, no randomized clinical trial with placebo-control consistently shows the anti-depressant benefits of VNS.

The VNS Neural Mechanism

The mechanism through which VNS will support non-common antidepressant patients is uncertain, and further research is required to explain this. Reports in functional neuroimaging have shown that VNS affects the behavior of many cortical and subcortical areas. The vagus nerve has systemic connections, via direct or indirect anatomic associations via the NTS, with several moods that control limbic and cortical brain areas.

For example, the PET scans in the chronic VNS for depression have shown a decrease in the brain rest in the ventromedial prefrontal cortex (vmPFC), which modulates the emotion in the amygdala and other brain regions. VNS may contribute to chemical changes in the synthesis of monoamine in these regions, which may lead to antidepressant action. Various types of research have shown the association between monoamine and antidepressant action. Each medication used in the synaptic cleft has antidepressant properties, which can increase monoamines — serotonin (5-HT), NE, or dopamine (DA). Depression of monoamines also contributes to depressive symptoms in individuals who have an elevated risk of depression.

Chronic VNS affects the brain and cerebrospinal fluid amounts of 5-HT, NE, and DA. In rats, VNS therapies have been shown to cause major, time-dependent changes in basal neuronal firing in the nucleus of the brainstem for serotonin in the dorsal raphe nucleus. Therefore, chronic VNS has been associated with increased extracellular levels of dorsal raphe serotonin.

Some evidence suggests that NE is a significant neurotransmitter in the treatment of pathophysiology and depressive disorders. The therapeutic loss of NE within the brain led to the restoration of depressive symptoms with NE antidepressant medications following successful treatment. The LC comprises the highest brain cell population and is estimated by NTS, which in turn is guided by the nerve vagus. Therefore, VNS decreases the firing rate of NE neurons and thus reduces the firing frequency of serotonin neurons. The NE abundance in the prefrontal cortex has thus been shown to increase. Disposal of noradrenergic neurons caused a loss of antidepressant VNS effects.

For AD, it has been shown that the short-term (14 days) and long-term effects (12 months) of VNS can contribute to dopaminergic activation in the brain stem. DA is a catecholamine that is synthesized widely in the gut and plays a decisive role in the brain's reward system.

In fact, the beneficial effects of VNS could be practiced monoamine-independent. Thus, VNS therapies may induce dynamic changes in the hippocampus of monoamine metabolites, and several studies have documented the impact of VNS on the neurogenesis of the hippocampus. This cycle was known to be a necessary biological process to maintain a normal mood.

Serotonin is a major neurotransmitter that can cause peristalsis and induce nausea and vomiting through the activation of the vagus nerve. Therefore, it is necessary to control important functions such as appetite and sleep and contributes to well-being feelings. At 95%, enterochromaffin cells are formed, a form of the neuroendocrine cell which lies next to the epithelium that lines the lumen of the digestive tract. Serotonin is released from enterochromaffin cells to mechanical or chemical gastrointestinal stimulation leading to 5-HT3 receptor activation on vagal afferent terminals. The vagal afferent neurons, including gastrointestinal vagal afferent neurons, are also found in 5-HT3 receptors, where they can be activated by 5-HT circulation. There are also 5-HT3 receptors at the central terminals of vagal afferents, which increase the glutamatergic synaptic transmission of nucleus tractus solitarius to second-order neurons in the brains. The relationships between vagus and serotonin processes in the intestine and brain also seem to play an important role in the management of psychiatric conditions.

VAGUS-RELATED DEPRESSION TREATMENT

Basic depression pathophysiology

A major depressive disorder is one of the leading causes of worldwide disease burden and mental health. The burden of unemployment is a major economic drain on our nation with a lifetime rate of 1.0 percent (Czech Republic) to 16.9 percent (US). Depression pathophysiology is diverse and includes social contextual stress factors, genetic and biological mechanisms such as HPA overdriving, inflammation, and monoamine neurotransmission disruptions, as mentioned above. A deficiency of amino acid tryptophan, which precedes serotonin, can, for example, cause depressive symptoms such as depressed mood, depression, and despair.

In subjects with severe depression (i.e., with melancholic or psychotic depression), the overdrive of the HPA axis is most frequently observed if the inhibitory mechanisms of cortisol are impaired that lead to cytokine oversealing. Chronic exposure to elevated inflammatory cytokines has been shown to contribute to depression. The fact that cytokine overexpression contributes to a decrease in serotonin levels may explain this. Therapy with anti-inflammatory drugs, therefore, has the potential to reduce depressive symptoms. As a result, IBD is a significant risk factor for mood and anxiety disorders, which increase the risk of IBD exacerbation.

Depression VNS

The positive effects of VNS in depressive symptoms have been shown in a European multicenter study of people with treatment-resistant depression. The deployment of VNS over a three-month period resulted in a response rate of 37% and a remission rate of 17%.

After 1 year of therapy, the response rate reached 53%, and the remission rate reached 33%. A meta-analytic analysis of VNS use in depressed patients revealed an acute illness response rate of about 50 percent and a long-term rescue rate of 20 percent after 2 years of treatment. In recurrent therapeutic resistant depression, several other studies also showed an increasing long-term benefit of VNS. Furthermore, a5-year prospective study evaluating the results of care as normal and of VNS as an adjunctive treatment only in drug-resistant depression showed better clinical outcomes and a higher rate of recovery in the VNS community. This was also the case with patients with comorbid depression and anxiety who often do not respond in antidepressant trials. All of these experiments were open-label and did not use a randomized, placebo-controlled method. It is important to note that

Patients of depression have elevated levels of proinflammatory cytokines in blood and cerebrospinal fluid. The advantage of VNS in depression could be because of an inhibitory effect in the development of proinflammatory cytokines and large peripheral rises in anti-inflammatory circulating cytokines. Additionally, improvements after VNS have been linked to altered CRH secretion and thus to prevent overdrive of the HPA axis. CRH production and secretion may result from direct stimulating effects transmitted to the paraventricular nucleus of the hypothalamus from the vagus nerve through NTS. VNS has also been shown to suppress peripheral TNF-α blood development in clinical depression.

Nutrition Influence Depressive symptoms

The intestinal microbiota is the main modulator of the immune systems and nervous systems. Targeting it could lead to an increase in the mental symptoms of stressed or nervous patients. Nutritional factors like probiotics, gluten, and medications such as antioxidants and antibiotics have growing effects on distinctly nervous function by contact with the gut microbiota, which varies greatly amongst individuals. However, animal studies have shown that microbiota contact with the brain includes the vagus nerve, and this connection can contribute to mediating brain and behavioral results.

Lactobacillus species, for example, have received tremendous attention as a result of their use as probiotics and health promoters. Several studies have shown that prolonged treatment of mice with Lactobacillus rhamnosus (strain B-1) decreased the levels of stress-induced corticosterone and triggered anxiety and depression. A chronic diagnosis of L has been shown. Caused spatial based changes in GABA(B1b) mRNA in the brain caused by rhamnose (jB-1), with raises in the cortical (singular and prelimbic) regions and parallel decreases in the hippocampus, amygdala, and LC function. Therefore, L. Rhamnosus (JB-1) decreased GABA(Aα2) mRNA expression in the prefrontal cortex and amygdala but increased the hippocampus GABA(Aα2), which balanced typical depressive symptoms pathogenesis, namely a lack of prefrontal regulation and overactivity of subcortical, nervous brain regions. Significantly, L. Rhamnosis (JB-1) decreased stress-inducing corticosterone and activity related to anxiety and depression. This is not unexpected as variations in the core expression of the GABA receptor are implicated in the pathogenesis of anxiety and depression. The fear and antidepressant effects of L. Among the vasectomized muzzle, the primary modulatory route of communication between the intestinal and brain exposed bacteria has not been identified as vagus. Accordingly, before colitis activation in Bifidobacterium longum therapy was absent, the anxiety effect in a chronic colitis paradigm associated with anxiety-like behavior in mice vasectomized.

Psychobiotics can be used in humans to treat patients with psychological problems by antidepressant and anxiolytic activity (133) in a genus of probiotics with anti-inflammatory properties. Differences in the makeup of intestinal microbiota in depressed patients have been shown in contrast with healthy individuals. Especially the fecal samples collected from five depressed patients transferred to germ-free mice have resulted in suicidal behavior.

Relaxation techniques affect depressive symptoms

It has been shown that self-generated positive emotions by loving-childhood meditation lead to an increase in positive emotions in comparison to the control group. In effect, increased positive emotions produced vagal tone changes, presumably influenced by increased social expectations. Persons of depression, anxiety, and chronic pain have undergone regular meditation instruction, which showed a dramatic improvement in the severity of the symptoms.

Controlled studies have found yoga-based approaches that are effective in treating depression, from minor depressive to major depressive (MDD) symptoms. Many yoga activities will specifically activate the vagus nerve by increasing the vagal tone to enhance self-regulation, cognitive functions, and mood and stress control. The suggested neurophysiological pathways for yoga-based treatments to relieve depressive symptoms suggest that breathing yoga causes vagal tone. Several experiments show the brain function and physiological conditions of yogic breathing. Therefore, the meditative meditation technique of Sudarshan Kriya Yoga (SKY) stimulates the vagus of the nerve and has numerous independent effects, including improvements in heart rate, increased memory, and improved bowel function. During the SKY, a series of different frequency, speed, volume, and end-inspire or end-expiratory breathing strategies produces a range of stimulus from numerous visceral afferents, sensory receptors, and baroreceptors. They probably affect different vagal fibers, which in turn lead to physiological changes in the liver and affect the limbial system. Recent studies have shown that even patients not responding to antidepressants have shown significant reductions in the symptoms of depression and anxiety compared to the control group following eight weeks of SKY adjunctive therapy.

For people with depression, Iyengar yoga was shown to reduce depressive symptoms. Iyengar yoga is associated with increased HRV, which reinforces the belief that yoga relaxation and postures function, in part, through increased parasympathy.

VAGUS-RELATED PTSD TREATMENT

PTSD pathophysiology

Chronic trauma is an anxiety disorder that may occur after trauma and is characterized by unwanted thoughts, hallucinations, hypervigilance, delusions, social avoidance, and social dysfunctions. It has an 8.3 percent lifespan prevalence using the DSM-5 definition. PTSD symptoms can be divided into four groups: disruption effects, behavior, cognitive and affective changes, and anxiety and behavioral changes. People with PTSD tend to live as if they are under constant threat. They show fighting and flight behavior, or a perpetual shutdown and dissociation, without the possibility of calming and developing positive social interactions. Through time, these independent maladaptive responses lead to increased risk of psychological comorbidities, such as alcohol and cardiovascular disease.

The signs of post-traumatic stress disorder are regulated in part by the vagus nerve. The reduced parasympathetic activity in PTSD is shown to suggest an independent discrepancy. The subtly regulated heart rate that myelinated vagal fibers vary with breathing. The vagal effect on the heart can, therefore, be measured by quantification of the amplitude of heart rate rhythmic fluctuations — respiratory sinus arrhythmia (RSA). A recent study found a decreased RSA rest in PTSD veterans. Furthermore, PTSD patients displayed a greater heart rate variation than healthy controls.

One of the many features of PTSD is the constant presentation of depressive responses of affected manifestations despite the absence of external stress. Behavioral treatments for PTSD focus on helping the patient raising their fear of this disorder over time. Exposure-based treatments are thus considered the gold standard in PTSD therapy. The goal of exposure-based therapy is to replace chronic trauma associations with new, more acceptable associations that contrast with fearful associations. Studies have demonstrated that PTSD patients have impaired memory extinction and defective activation of the network of terror extinction. The vmPFC, amygdala, and hippocampus are part of this network. It is very important for the theoretical retrieval of experiences of anxiety following extinction.

The signs of frequency and anatomical defects in the anterior hippocampus and centromedian amygdala have been linked with posttraumatic stress disorder. There is evidence of increased amygdala activity during programmed fear in humans and rodents. The amygdala and vmPFC have reciprocal synaptic connections. Indeed, PFC can be hypoactive under conditions of uncertainty and threat and can not inhibit the overactivity of the amygdala with the appearance of PTSD symptoms, such as hyperarousal and re-experience. In comparison, PTSD-patients have shown increased activation of the basolateral amygdala during involuntary facial perception relative to healthy controls and patients with panic disorders and generalized anxiety disorders in response to emotional experiences as frightening expressions.

The hippocampus is also an essential component of the fear circuit and is involved in PTSD pathophysiology. Patients of PTSD display decreased concentration of the hippocampus, consistent with the severity of the symptoms. The hippocampus is a central organ for temporal processing and episodic memory. Hippocampal disruption contributes to deficiencies in human and rodent background decoding. The neural circuit consisting of the hippocampus, amygdala, and vmPFC is of major importance for the contextual collection of fear memories following extinction. Impairment of the hippocampal functioning and the resulting generalization of dysfunctional context in PTSD patients may cause patients to experience symptoms related to trauma again.

PTSD VNS

Vagus nerve stimulation has proven promising in treatment-resistant anxiety disorders, including PTSD, as a therapeutic option. Chronic VNS has shown that anxiety in rats is minimized, and the Hamilton anxiety score is improved in people who have behavioral resistant depression. The vagus nerve transmits signals to the NTS and the NTS transmits direct projections to the amygdala and hypothalamus. In fact, VNS stimulates NE activation in the basolateral amygdala as well as the hippocampus and cortex. NE amygdala infusion contributes to better extinction understanding. VNS could, therefore, be a good tool for increasing preservation in biodiversity. For example, extinction combined with VNS therapy in rats can lead to anxiety recovery and changes in PTSD-like symptoms. Further, VNS in combination with extinction learning facilitates plasticity between the infralimbic media prefrontal cortex and the basolateral amygdala complex in order to enable the extinction of conditioned fear reactions. Therefore, VNS can boost survival by inhibiting the sympathetic nervous system function. An immediate reduction in anxiety caused by VNS can contribute to VNS-led extinction by interfering with the sympathetic CS reaction and thus disrupting the association between CS and fear.

Randomized controlled trials are, however, mandatory to support these findings.

One of the most consistent neurophysiological effects of VNS is to decrease hippocampal activity by increasing GABAergic signaling. The hippocampus is, as described, a crucial part of the fear circuit because it is a major structure for episodic memory and spatial context encoding. Decreased hippocampal activity following VNS in a number of other studies was reported in other conditions such as depression or schizophrenia.

The positive influence of PTSD nutrients

Emerging research suggests that probiotics can decrease inflammatory responses due to stress as well as associated symptoms. An exploratory analysis investigating the microbiota of patients with PTSD and of trauma-exhibited controls showed that in PTSD patients with higher PTDS symptoms, the presence of three strains was reduced: Actinobacteria, Lentisphaerae, and Verrucomicrobia. Such bacteria are critical for immune control, and their decreased abundance may lead to immune system dysregulation and the development of PTSD symptoms. Research using a murine PTSD model found that immunization with the heat-killed immunoregulatory bacteria Mycobacterium vaccine (NCTC 11659) has contributed to a more positive behavioral response to psychosocial stress. Research in healthy volunteers has shown that the administration of various probiotics has been related to greater well-being and a decrease in anxiety and psychological distress. All of these findings are unofficial. Well-designed, double-blind, placebo-controlled clinical trials are desperately necessary to determine the impact of bacterial supplementation and controlled dietary modification on psychological symptoms and cognitive functions in PTSD patients.

Positive meditation and yoga effects on PTSD

The efficacy of consciousness-based stress reduction (MBSR) in the management of PTSD has clinical evidence. Slow breathing and long breathing periods lead to an increase in the parasympathetic tone during MBSR. However, clinical trials have shown that yoga is effective as a therapeutic intervention for PTSD and dissociation by reducing the stress response. Yoga also decreases the effects of PSTD after natural disasters. Yoga-responsive anxiety disorders, including PTSD, incorporate higher HRV and low GABA. The PFC, Hippocampus, and Amygdala connections, together with the autonomous nervous system and GABA inputs, are a network through which yoga-based activities can decrease symptoms. There is evidence that the reduced vmPFC regulation of the amygdala function is correlated with a compromised regression from programmed fear in PTSD. PFC activation linked to increased parasympathetic activity during yoga can enhance amygdala inhibition through PFC GABA projections, reduce the overactivity of the amygdala, and reduce PTSD symptoms.

VAGUS-RELATED WITH INFLAMMATORY TREATMENT DISEASE

IBD Pathophysiology

Inflammatory bowel disease mainly consists of two disorders: Colitis ulcerative (UC) and Crohn's disease (CD). IBD is characterized by persistent, unregulated inflammation of the intestinal mucosa. Abdominal pain, diarrhea, fever, weight loss, and extra-intestinal (skin, hair, joints) signs are typical of the symptoms. Diarrhea, abdominal pain, and weight loss are the primary symptoms on CD, while UC diarrhea is the main symptom, frequently followed by rectal bleeding.

Inflammatory bowel disease affects about 1.5 million people in the United States and 2.2 million people in

Europe, and around 20 percent of IBD patients have a successful family history. Therefore, industrialization has led to significant changes in the prevalence of IBDs in Asia. There is increasing evidence of environmental risk factors, including illness, western diet, and food additives, air, and water contamination, medication (antibiotics, hormones) and genetic factors (more than 250 genetic factors were reliably identified), which contribute in time to an irregular immune response to microbial exposure. What differentiates IBD from inflammatory responses seen in the normal intestines is the inability to de-regulate inflammatory reactions like when the intestines get inflamed as a result of a possible disease pathogen.

Thus, the mucosal immune system remains chronically activated and chronically inflamed in individuals with IBD inflammation. The cytokines (IL-1β,IL-6, TNF-α) that come out of the intestinal mucosa activate VN afferents, which end in the NTS during inflammation, then relay visceral information to the activation of the HPA axis. In addition, the anti-inflammatory function of vagus efferents was reported through the CAIP. As previously noted, the development of proinflammation cytokines such as TNF-α is decreased by ACh produced at the distal end of VN efferents. The exaggeration of the TNF-α may be a crucial step in the development of IBD.

IBD VNS

Stimulation of the vagus nerves decreases the systemic inflammatory response of endotoxins and intestinal inflammation. The VNs also modulate the immune response of the spleen indirectly through interacting with the splenic sympathetic nerve. In colonized rats, the 3-hour average VNS for five days resulted in lower inflammatory factors and better colitis symptoms.

Other inflammatory diseases, such as rheumatoid arthritis, another TNF-α-medicated disease, should be of interest in vagus nerve stimulation. A study in patients with rhcumatoid arthritis showed improvements in early and late phases of 1–4 minutes of VNS a day. The first study showed that VNS prevents the development of TNF-α and other cytokines in humans by activating the inflammatory mirror and reducing the severity of the symptoms. These results advocate for the vagus nerve's anti-inflammatory function and provide possible therapeutic uses for patients with IBDs.

Positive nutrient impact on IBD

Through function, greater attention has been paid to the role of inflammation in the appearance and perpetuation of psychiatric symptoms. The increase in dysfunctionality in modern urban societies was at least partly linked to decreased exposure to commensal and environmental micro-organisms that normally prime immunoregulatory circuits and prevent improper inflammation. Bacterial flora of the intestines is considered a major factor in the progression and recurrence of IBD, and several attempts were made to alter flora with probiotics.

Improvements have been observed in animals with untreated colitis administered orally or rectally. Lactobacillus Plantarum 299V, for example, avoided disease onset and reduced developed colitis. Furthermore, the probiotic multi-species (VSL no. 3) given to mice with normalized colitis bowel function, reduced proinflammatory cytokines, and reduced histologic illness. Lactobacillus casei GG improved symptoms in humans in children with moderately active CD. In fact, there were slight improvements in the symptoms of CD with a mixture of probiotics, including Saccharomyces boulardii, Lactobacillus, and VSL#3. Such results are provisional and require additional analyses to validate. Several probiotic therapies for the diagnosis of CD have so far been formally approved.

In UC, clear evidence is provided that VSL#3 is useful for the treatment of mildly infected pouchitis. E. Coli Nissle, part of VSL#3, can be as effective in sustaining remission as mesalamine.

IBD Hypnotherapy, Meditation, and Yoga Positive influence An increasing number of studies have shown the benefits of IBD therapeutic treatment. For example, a randomized controlled trial of a calming therapy technique in conjunction with a control group showed reductions in discomfort, decreased anxiety levels, and improved quality of life. Additionally, treatment based on empathy, a systematic mind-body plan, exercise, complementary mental-body approaches, yoga, and relaxation-based mental-body therapies has proved effective for IBD patients. In addition, vagal tone hypnotherapy has been effective in IBD treatment.

WHY THE VAGUS NERVE IS SO IMPORTANT

When my husband passed away, my depression was so serious that I tried to reduce it from dietary treatments to energy healing. In a moment I cannot recall, the energy healer I met said, "The central nervous system is fried, and I am so worried about you." So it might seem a little "out there" and woo-woo for someone, but this lady has helped me cure so many of the things I was struggling with and telling her that she is concerned about a part of my body that I had been full otherwise. I didn't know that there was a nervous system at heart, and I still find today that few people know how to relax or stimulate it properly.

The vagus nerve (pronounced Vegas) regulates so many important functions in your body from breathing to the heartbeat, which can act as a "hack" to the right health when adequately stimulated. Problems with your central nervous system often go unnoticed, because you may not sense them immediately, or they can occur in several forms, like through your intestines or your brain. This is the reason that this nerve is so vital–you can improve your health and fix any complications before they start to develop by finding ways to keep it working properly.

What is this little-known about, and how can you use it for your health? Why is the vagus nerve so important?

The vagus nerve may be one of the least known, but also one of the body's most significant nerves. It plays a part in so many vital functions of our body, from the "rest and digestion" of our parasympathetic nervous system to our sympathetic nervous system's "fight or flight" reaction. The nerve travels from the brain through the neck and belly to the colon–allowing sensory information to be conveyed throughout the body.

This nerve is not only linked to our regular daily functions such as cardiac velocity, breathing, and memories but also plays a major role in one of the wellness topics most spoken of today–the gut. Essentially, the vagus nerve will detect the bacteria in your gut and transmit tactile feedback and information to the central nervous system.

So what does that mean exactly?

That your brain and intestines are really connected, and the vagus nerve is the key contact point between the two. Therefore, if you are nervous, you can have an upset stomach or some issues in your bathroom–

discomfort hinders the vagus nerve that can remove the digestive system and lead to problems such as IBS and IBD (inflammatory bowel disease). Nevertheless, if the vagus is agitated, it can induce much-needed homeostasis in the stomach.

How can the vagus nerve be supported?

If your vagus nerve is properly stimulated and operated, it can do incredible things for your body. Studies show that vagus nerve stimulation can have anti-depressant, anti-inflammatory, digestive, brain-improving effects, and so many more! But how do you benefit from the boosts in health that a properly stimulated vagus nerve can bring? Here are some ways:

Deep breathing– A 2010 study revealed that slow abdominal participants had improved vagal nerve activity. Try to lie on your abdomen in a comfortable place. Breathe in and keep it for a couple of seconds, imagine the air flooding your uterus and gradually flowing through your teeth. At least 10 minutes per day follow these steps.

Intermittent fasting–Studies indicate that intermittent fasting activates the vagus nerve rather than only a food phenomenon.

Taking probiotics–We have already discussed how to give thanks for the unique intestinal connection to the vagus nerve, but certain bacterial and nutritional stimuli (such as probiotics) can enhance the nerve and the signals it sends.

Show compassion–This is certainly something we must always do, but being pleased and caring towards others can also have some personal benefits, especially for this vital nerve. Compassion can not only activate the vagus nerve by the brain, but even more often are people who have an activated and stimulated vagus nerve–it's a loop that makes you feel good for yourself and others!

Practice Yoga –Regular yoga exercises will activate the vagus nerve and improve the performance of your sympathetic system, contributing to improved mood, energy, and cardiac function.

ANATOMY OF VAGUS NERVE

Vagus nerve (CN X, also known as the vagus, Latin: nervus vagus) is the most widely spread cranial nervous system in the human body, as it spans not only forms in the brain but also runs through the spine, thorax, and abdomen, supplying a number of visceral organs.

The vagus nerve is a combined nerve with somatic and visceral fibers and normal and special visceral efferent fibers.

The vagus nerve fibers originate from 3 nuclei:

• nucleus ambiguous,

• Vagus nerve dorsal nucleus

• The nucleus of the solitary tract

The ambiguous nuclide consists of motor-neuron bodies that generate unique visceral efferent fibers that provide innervation for branch-arch skeletal muscles such as the muscular cricothyroid, pharynx muscles, and intrinsic larynx muscles.

The vagus nerve's dorsal nucleus comprises general visceral efferent nerves, which provide the viscera with parasympathetic innervation.

The solitary tract nucleus (also referred to as the solitary tract nucleus) comprises neurons that receive information from specific afferent visceral fibers that carry sensory information from the epiglottis, and general afferent visceral fibers which transmit sensory information from the soft palate mucosa, pharynx, and larynx.

It can be separated into cranial, cervical, thoracic, and abdominal elements.

Cranial Vagus Nerve Component

Rootlets from the medulla oblongata form smaller, lower and lower upper bundles that collectively form the vagus nerve after leaving the medulla, along with the glossy-pharyngeal nerve (CN IX), and the cranial root of the supplementary nerve (CN XI). The vagus nerve is followed by the peripheral nerve through the jugular foramen, all of them with arachnoids and a dural sheath. The upper (jugular) and lower (nodose) ganglions below the jugular foramen of the vagus nerve, where pseudounipolar neurons are located, have two enlargements.

The upper vagus nerve ganglion contains afferent somatosensory neuronal cells. Many axons lead to a branch of the vagus nerve, which provides sensory information from the external auditory tissue, the auricular nerve. Many fibers form the meningeal branch of the vagus nerve in the cranial fossa posterior to the raw mother, while a number of fibers transmit impulses from the epiglottis and vallecular epiglottis of the flavor receptors.

The lower ganglion of the vagus nerve comprises somatic, unique, and general visceral afferent neurons with axons centrally synaptic in the solitary nucleus and their dendrites that obtain sensory data in the section of the larynx, pulm, heart and food tract from the pharynx to the transverse colon.

Vagus Nerve Cervical Part

Upon entering the skull through the jugular foramen, the vagus nerve descends to the neck of the carotid sheath between the inner carotid artery and the inner juvenile vein, and from the outer carotid artery to the inner jugular vein.

Four collections of branches arise in the cervical portion of the vagus nerve:

• pharyngeal branches

• Bottom laryngeal nerve

• Laryngeal nerve recurring

• Heart divisions

The vagus nerve's pharyngeal branches are found in the upper part of the lower vagal ganglion and contain filaments that also form the accessory nerve (CN XI). On the neck, pharyngeal branches of the vagus migrate through external and inner carotid arteries to the upper limit of the middle pharyngeal constrictor and are stretched into several filaments that join branches of the sympathetic cord and glossopharyngeal nerve (CN IX). Together with the peripheral nerve, the pharyngeal nerve plexus is used to intervals the pharyngeal (except the CN IX-internalizing stylopharyngeal, mucus membrane in the lower part of the pharynx, and sensitive palate muscles (except the CN V3-internalized tensor veli palatini).

The upper laryngeal nerve is a vagus nerve branch with both sensory and motor fibers. The upper laryngeal nerve arises from the middle of the lower ganglion of the vagus nerve, and in its course, is divided into internal and external branches of the laryngeal nerve by a branch of the upper cervical sympathetic Ganglion and then moved alongside the pharynx to the inner carotid artery. The inner branch of the top laryngeal nerve provides the pharynx with sensory internalization, but the exterior branch of the top laryngeal nerve contains motor fibers that interview the cricothyroid muscle.

The recurrent laryngeal nerve is a mixed motor-and sensory-fibreated branch of the vagus nerve. The recurrent laryngeal nerve varies from left and right in frequency and direction. The word' recurrent' suggests that they move in the opposite direction towards the nerve from which they branch. On the left side, the recurrent laryngeal nerve loops underneath the aortic ark, while the right nerve loops below the first part of the right subclavian artery, and both nerves at this point give the deeper cardiac plexus a cardiac filament. After that, laryngeal nerves climb tightly to the medial surface of the thyroid gland above the groove between the esophagus and the trachea and then pass into the lower edge of a constrictive muscle, passing into the larynx. The repeated motor fibers of the laryngeal nerve cycles all but the cricothyroid laryngeal muscles. It also interacts with the laryngeal nerve and provides the laryngeal mucosa with (afferent) tactile fibers under the vocal folds as well as with afferent fibers from the laryngeal stretch receptors.

The vagus nerve has two pairs of cardiac branches, the higher and the lower cervical cardiac branches.

The lower cervical cardiac branches of the vagus are triggered by the vagus nerve, the vagus nerve on the right side, the vaginal nerve trunk, and the recurrent laryngeal nerve, while the recurrent nerve on the right side is only formed. The lower cervical heart branches descend to the deep segment of the cardiac plexus behind subclavius arthritis and along the front of the trachea.

The upper cervical core branches of the vagus nerve emerge from the upper cervical ganglion as two branches. They run down behind the common carotid artery and cross the long collar muscle and the recurrent laryngeal nerve before the lower thyroid artery. The right branch is associated with the deep part of the heart plexus, while the left branch is running across the left and the left artery of the aorta to enter the shallow portion of the heart plexus.

In fact, the position of the vagus nerve on both sides varies. The right vagus nerve goes back to the juvenile vein, which runs through the first portion of the subclavian artery, which exits the lungs through the upper chest aperture. On the left, the vagus nerve joins in the thorax between the left popular artery and the brachiocephalic arteries.

Thoracic Vagus Nerve Part

The left and right vagus nerves run behind both the pulmonary radius and around the core of the esophagus in the thorax, and the fibers converge to form the esophageal plexus. The lower fibers of the esophageal plexus form the vagal trunks before and after. The anterior vagal trunk sheds fibers on the anterior esophagus floor. This consists mainly of left vagus fibers. The posterior vagal trunk is mainly made up of fibers from the right vagus nerve and is spread over the rear surface of the esophagus. All trunks descend into the abdominal cavity through the esophageal gap in the diaphragm.

Abdominal Vagus Nerve Part

The anterior vagus is divided in the abdomen along the lower curvature of the stomach into several branches: the anterior gastric branches which form the anterior gastric plexus and supply the stomach;

the hepatic branch which moves along the lower momentum to the liver; the celiac branch, which is composed of small branches which provide parasympathetic innervation to the heart This posterior vagal trunk is separated in several divisions by the greater curvature of the stomach up to the posterior surface:

the posterior gastric branches, which are the anterior gastric plexus, kidney branches, liver and gallbladder branches, and the celiac branch of the celiac nerve plexus, which contain almost all the abdominal organs.

9 FASCINATING FACTS ABOUT THE VAGUS NERVE

The vagus nerve is so-called because it "walks" like a vagabond and transmits sensory fibers to your visceral organs from your brainstem. The vagus, the largest of the cranial nerves, regulates the core of your inner nerve— the parasympathetic nervous system. This controls a wide range of key functions, sending motor and sensory signals to each organ in your body. New research has shown that the missing link with the treatments of serious, incurring diseases and the beginning of an exciting new thérapeutic field is chronic inflammation. There are nine facts concerning this powerful bundle of nerves here.

1. The vagus ' nerve prevents inflammation

Upon injury or disease, a certain level of inflammation is common. But there are many diseases and conditions associated with an overabundance, from sepsis to the autoimmune state of rheumatoid arthritis. The vagus nerve has a huge fiber network deployed around all the tissue-like spies. This alerts the brain and pulls out anti-inflammatory neurotransmitters that control the body's immune response when the warning is received for incipient inflammation— the production of cytokines or a substance called a tumor necrosis factor (TNF).

2. It allows you to remember

Research by the University of Virginia in rats has shown that their vagus nerves activate their memory. The activity transferred the norepinephrine neurotransmitter into the hippocampus, consolidating memories. Similar human studies have shown potential therapies for disorders such as Alzheimer's disease.

3. It will allow you to relax

The acetylcholine neurotransmitter released by the vagus nerve allows the lungs to breathe. This is one of the reasons that Botox –often used cosmetically–may be harmful, as it inhibits the development of acetylcholine. Nevertheless, you can also activate the vagus nerve by respiring or breathing in 4 to 8 counts.

4. With your head, it is closely involved

The vagus nerve regulates the heart rate through electrical impulses to a specific muscular tissue— the normal pacemaker of the heart— in the right atrium, where the release of acetylcholine slows down the heartbeat. If you calculate the interval between each actual pulse and map this overtime on a monitor, doctors will assess the amplitude of your heart rate or HRV. This data can provide insights into the strength of your heart and vagus nerve.

5. It initiates your body's response to relaxation

If your ever-watching sympathetic nervous system works around to fight and flight reactions— spreading adrenaline and adrenalin into your bloodstream — the vagus nerve advises the body to reset itself by releasing acetylcholine. The vagus nerve sinews stretch through many tissues, functioning as fiber-optic cables, which give signals to activate prolactin, vasopressin, and oxytocin enzymes and proteins, which will calm you down. Individuals with stronger vagus responses can recover faster from stress, injury, or disease.

6. Among your positive and your soul

The intestines use the vagus nerve like a walkie-talkie to inform the subconscious how you feel through electrical impulses known as "acting power." The intestinal sensation is true. 7 Overstimulation of the vagus nerve is the most common source of fainting. When you tremble or get queasy when you see blood or get a flu shot, you are not tired.

WAYS TO UNLOCK THE POWERS OF THE VAGUS NERVE

How to pull up your nervous system

The vagus nerve is probably the most important nerve you didn't know about.

Everything that occurs in this vagus does not linger there, unlike the other Vegas. The obscure nerve is an organ and a tactile body that meanders long and links the brain's nucleus to the heart, lungs, and stomach. Also branching are the liver, spleen, gallbladder, ureter, feminine fertility, organs, neck, ears, tongue & kidneys. It enhances our subconscious nervous system-part sympathy-center by maintaining a stable feeding rhythm by breathing and sweating, controlling the involuntary functions of the body. It also supports the blood pressure and glucose balance, promotes renal function overall, helps the release of bile and testosterone, promotes saliva secretion and helps to control taste and release tears.

Dr. Justin Hoffman, a Santa Rosa, California licensed naturopathic physician, says:

• The key functions that keep us alive are not preserved without vagus nervousness.

Brandon Mentore is a nationally renowned sports nutritionist, strength specialist, and conditioner:

• The Vagus Nerve is extremely important for your overall health and is closely related to multiple organ and cell functions.

The vagus nerve has fibers, which essentially inside all our inner organs. Emotional control and absorption take place via the vagal nerve between the heart, brain, and intestines, which is why we have a good intestinal response against extreme mental and emotional states.

Vagus nerve dysfunction may result in a variety of conditions including hypertension, bradycardia (abnormally slow heartbeat), swallowing problems, gastrointestinal disorders, fainting, anxiety, B12 deficiency, excessive vomiting, cough loss, and convulsion.

While the activation of the vagus nervous system has been shown to improve conditions such as:

- Anxiety disorder
- Heart disease

- Tinnitus
- Obesity
- Alcohol addiction
- Migraines
- Alzheimer's
- Leaky gut
- Bad blood circulation
- Mood disorder
- Cancer

Look closer to this incredible nerve

The vagus nerve is our 12 cranial nerves ' longest. Only the heart is a larger nervous system. Approximately 80% of its nerve fibers, or 4 of its five' lanes,' carry input from the body to the brain. The fifth lane runs in the opposite direction and shuts signals across the entire body from the brain. The vagus is rooted in the brain stem, separated by the neck and the shoulders into the left vagus and the right vagus. Every path has tens of thousands of nerve fibers that branch into the heart, lung, liver, pancreas, and almost every other organ in the abdomen.

The vagus nerve uses the acetylcholine neurotransmitter, which induces contractions of muscles in the parasympathetic nervous system. A neurotransmitter is a kind of chemical messenger released at the end of a nerve fiber, which permits signals to move from point to point, stimulating different organs. Of starters, if the release of acetylcholine from the vagus nerve could not interact with our brain, then we would stop breathing.

Many substances, such as botox and heavy metal mercury, may interfere with acetylcholine development. Botox is believed to shut down the vagus nerve, leading to death. Mercury prevents acetylcholine activity. When mercury is bound to thiol protein in the heart muscle receptors, the vagus nerve electrical signal for contraction can not be transmitted by the heart muscles. Usually, cardiovascular complications priced. The mercury used in fillings from the brain just inches, and the 3,000 tons of mercury deposited in the atmosphere that interfere with the development of acetylcholine. In vague childhood autism related to nerves, mercury-laden vaccines could also play a role.

Hoffman says: He says:

• In principle, anything that helps to improve acetylcholine's existence and function will also help to reduce the health of our vagus nerve.

He suggests natural nootropic huperzine and galantamine enhance receptor sensitivity.

Diabetes, alcoholism, upper respiratory viral infections, or severe accidental part of the nerve during operation can also result in damage to the vagus nerve. Stress and exhaustion and fear will inflame the nerve. Such an easy as a poor posture can have a negative effect on the vagus nerve.

Diet is also known to play a role in the health of vagus nerves. A high fat, high-carbon' cafeteria diet ' reduces the vulnerability of the vagus nerve. Spicy foods can also confuse them.

Feeling in your goodness

The acupuncturist and practitioner of Oriental and spiritual health, Dr. Mark Sircus, says that people say they have felt this in their hearts.

Our intestines are real signs of nervousness that guide our lives, not imaginations.

This is because the entry nervous system (ENS), which controls the function of the gastrointestinal tract, communicates with the central nervous system (brain) through the vagus nervous system. This is considered the digestive brain pole. The ENS is sometimes called the second brain or replacement brain in our solar plexus. We now know that the ENS is not just autonomous, but controls the brain. Sircus continues: Indeed, about 90% of the signals that pass the vagus nerve do not come from above, but from the ENS.

The good condition of the stomach and vagus nerve channel impacts our mental health. A recent study shows how antibiotics can make us aggressive if they disrupt our gut's microbiome balance. Essential research by McMaster University in Hamilton, Ontario, Canada last year found that some helpful intestinal bacteria can prevent PTSD. Probiotic products will help to maintain gut and vague signals in a healthy state, according to the NBI (National Center for Biotechnology Information).

In Glenview, Illinois, Dr. Abby Kramer, holistic physician, and chiropractor explains:

• Probiotics help promote distinctly healthy action by its relation to the intestines and digestive functions. Zinc is also an excellent addition to people with stress or mental health problems and is also related to the vague nerve.

Electricity boosting

Doctors have long taken advantage of the influence of the nerve on the brain. Electric stimulation of the vagus nerve is sometimes used to treat people with epilepsy or depression, known as the Vagus Nerve Stimulation (VNS). VNS is designed to prevent seizures with normal, gentle electrical pulses sent to the brain through the vagus nerve. Such bursts are provided by a pacemaker-like system. It is placed below the skin on the wall of the chest, and a wire runs from it into the vagus nerve in the neck. Studies who studied the effects of vagus stimulation on epilepsy found that patients had a second advantage that was not linked to seizure reduction: they also changed moods.

A study published in 2016 in the Proceedings from the national academy of sciences (PNAS), revealed the significantly improved calculation of disease occurrence in individuals with rheumatoid arthritis, persistent inflammatory disease affecting 0.2 million U.S. people and costing tens of trillions of dollars annually, in the stimulation of the vagus nerve with a bioelectronic tool.

12 Nerve Vagus relaxation methods

The vagus nerve must not be shocked to form. Similar to a muscle, it can also be toned and reinforced. Here are some simple things you can do that will greatly improve your health:

1. Personal Relationships Good –.

A study showed people compassionately worrying about others while passively repeating optimistic statements about friends and families. In contrast to monitors, after finishing the training, the meditators have shown an overall increase in positive emotions such as calm, happiness, and hope. These positive thinking of others led to an improvement in vaguely functioned variability of the heart rate. The tests also showed a toned vagus nerve rather than just meditating.

2. Cold–"Hot treatment like cold showers or facial dunking activates the nerve," Mentore said.

Studies show that when the body adapts to freezing, your combat system decreases, or your flight system (sympathetic), and that your rest and digestion (parasympathetic) increases — and that vagus nerve mediates. Some form of acute cold exposure like drinking ice cold water increases the stimulation of the vagus nerves.

3. Gargling – Gargling of water is another home remedy for the under-stimulated vagus nerve. Yes, gargling activates the pallet muscles activated by the vagus nerve.

"We usually recommend that patients tear up a bit, and if they don't, we suggest that they do it consistently every day until they feel that they are tearing up a little," says Hoffman. "It was shown to boost working memory efficiency automatically."

4. Singing and Chating –Singing, mantra chanting, hymn singing, and energetic singing all increase the varying heart rates. Singing is simply like beginning a vagal pump that sends calm waves. Singing on the top of your lungs serves to activate your vagus through muscles in the back of your throat. Singing in harmony, often performed in churches and synagogues, often improves the work of HRV and vagus. Singing has been found to increase oxytocin because it makes people feel closer to each other.

5. Massage–By massaging your feet and neck along the carotid sinus on either side of your body, along the carotid arteries, you can relax the vagus nerve. A neck massage can help to reduce convulsions. A foot massage can help lower your blood pressure and your heart rate. The vagus nerve can also be stimulated by a pressure massage. Such messages can help children gain weight by improving intestinal activity, primarily by manipulating the vagus nerve.

6. Laughter–normal immunity boosters are joy and laughter. Laughter also stimulates the nerve of the vagus. Research shows how laughter in a group environment increases HRV.

There are various cases of laughter weaning, and this may be so triggered by the vagus nerve / parasympathy mechanism. Fainting and urination, vomiting, coughing, or bowel movement are likely during laughing–all of which are helped by slightly triggering.

7. Yoga and Tai Chi — Both increase the activity of the vagus nerve and the parasympathetic system. Studies have shown that yoga increases GABA, which calms your brain's neurotransmitter. Researchers believe it does so through "fibers," which increase parasympathetic nervous system activity. For those who deal with anxiety or depression, this is particularly helpful.

Studies show that tai chi can also "transform vagal synchronization."

8. Deep and Quick Breathing — The heart and neck include neurons with receptors called baroreceptors that sense blood pressure and send neuronal signals to your brain. It reduces blood pressure and pulse rhythm by strengthening the vagus nerve. Slow respiration, with a respiratory time of approximately equal duration, increases the sensitivity of baroreceptors and vagal stimulation. Approximately 5-6 breathes per minute in the average adult may be very effective.

9. Exercise –Exercise increases the growth hormone of your brain, strengthens mitochondria in your brain, and helps reverse cognitive decline. But the vagus nerve, which contributes to positive brain and mental health effects, has also been shown to stimulate. Current activity frequently activates the vagus nerve regulated intestine surge.

10. Coffee Enemas-- Enemas are like sprints for your vagus nerve. In the procedure, the liver cleanse itself as it launches the poisonous bile into the little, then big, intestinal tract for evacuation. By maintaining the coffee 12 to 15 minutes, the blood will flow 4 to 5 times for cleaning, much like a dialysis treatment.

11. Nervana-- This wearable device stimulates a slight electrical pulse through the left ear canal to stimulate the vagus nerve in the body and to synchronize it with the music that activates neurotransmitters in the brain, to generate an extremely calming body experience.

12. Unwind-- The first thing that helps keep the vagus nerve toned could be to learn how to relax. According to Hoffman, the vagus nerve is activated by most cooperative practices.

- Eventually, this is where the most exceptionally felt effects can be discovered. Checking out a book, listening to music, enjoying kids' play-- whatever it is, my recommendations is to look for relaxation and make time in your life for it. ~ Dr. Justin Hoffman.

PLACEMENT, PROGRAMMING, AND SAFETY OF VAGUS NERVE STIMULATION (VNS)

How is the VNS gadget put?

Putting a vagus nerve stimulator can be performed in an outpatient setting. Here's a fast introduction of what to anticipate.

- The surgical treatment does NOT include opening the skull or operating on the brain in any method.
- The treatment is normally done under basic anesthesia. This implies you would be offered medication to make you go to sleep. You will not know what occurs throughout the surgical treatment.
- The cosmetic surgeon initially makes a cut on the left side of the chest. It is generally above the breast, along the external side of the chest, or under the left arm.
- The generator is then positioned under the skin. The generator is a thin, flat gadget.
- A 2nd cut is made on the left side of the neck, typically in the folds of the skin, so the scar is not seen later on.
- The stimulator electrode cable is wrapped on the left side of the neck around the vagus nerve.

- Once the electrode is put, it is threaded or put under the skin and connected to the generator.
- The treatment normally takes about 60 to 90 minutes.
- Usually, the individual goes house later on the exact same day.
- Often you might require to remain overnight in the healthcare facility for observation.

How is the VNS set?

The settings can be configured and altered by putting a wand over the generator on the left side of the chest. A cordless shows wand is utilized with the SenaTivaTM design of VNS.

- The SenTivaTM design can be set to immediately make modifications every 2 weeks without pertaining to the center. These modifications can be set up to take place as much as 7 times in the house, prior to the individual requires to come back for a see.
- The gadget is configured to go on (offer stimulation) for a specific duration (for instance, 7 seconds to 30 seconds) and after that to go off (stop stimulation) for another duration (for instance, 20 seconds to 5 minutes). The gadget is set to offer

stimulation at routine periods throughout the day and night.

- Settings (likewise called stimulation specifications) set by the company likewise consist of the output existing, signal frequency, and pulse width.
- The more recent designs can be configured to provide stimulation immediately in action to a modification in heart rate (called auto stimulation). When the auto stimulation needs to be provided and for how long, the developer will set.
- Changing various settings can enhance how the stimulation is endured and how well it works.

How is the VNS magnet utilized?

Everyone who has a VNS gadget is offered a set of magnets. These can be utilized to stop a seizure or to switch off the VNS briefly.

When a seizure occurs, the individual feeling the seizure or somebody who sees it can swipe the magnet. This might assist stop the seizure, make it much shorter, or less extreme.

To Stop A Seizure:

- Swipe the magnet over the generator in the left chest location for one second.
- Typically counting one-one thousand while it's swiped works well to ensure you are doing it properly.
- Some individuals might not have the ability to utilize the magnet, which's alright. Simply think about the magnet as an additional method of utilizing the VNS.
- Each time the magnet is swiped in this manner, an additional burst of stimulation is offered.
- Ensure you teach others how to utilize the magnet and make it a regular part of your seizure emergency treatment strategies.

To Turn The VNS Gadget Off:

- If negative effects from the stimulation are an issue, you can tape the magnet over the generator in the left chest location. This will switch off the stimulation briefly.
- As long as the magnet is kept over the generator, no stimulation will be offered.
- Once the magnet is gotten rid of, the generator will provide stimulation once again.

- When to utilize the magnet to turn off stimulation, - Talk to your health care group about.
- In some cases, individuals utilize the magnet to turn the VNS gadget off prior to they have a test or surgical treatment.
- Other times individuals might turn it off throughout specific activities.

What are the most typical adverse effects of vagus nerve stimulation?

Negative effects of VNS Treatment can be separated into 2 kinds: 1) those associated with the positioning of the gadget, and 2) negative effects that might occur with stimulation.

Surgical Treatment Adverse Effects

- After surgical treatment, there might be some pain or discomfort around the injuries for a couple of days.
- There is a little danger of infection of the injuries.
- Everybody ought to be provided clear directions on how to look after the injury and dressings after surgical treatment. Ask for checking out the nurse to inspect on the injuries throughout the very first

1-2 weeks if somebody lives alone or requires assistance inspecting the dressings.

- Any indications of infection after surgical treatment (such as excessive soreness, drain, bleeding from the injury, or fever) need to be reported to the cosmetic surgeon immediately. An antibiotic will be provided if required.
- If an infection is not dealt with quickly, the gadget might require to be gotten rid of.
- There is a really low danger of a nerve to the singing cables being impacted or extended throughout the surgical treatment. If this occurs, the singing cable on the side of surgical treatment might not work typically.
- Similar to any surgical treatment, an extremely little number of individuals might have difficulty with anesthesia. If you have actually had any issues with other surgical treatments, talk to your physician.

Negative Effects of Configuring and Stimulation

The most typical negative effects seen with stimulation consist of:

- Hoarseness or modification in speech pattern
- Cough
- Amusing sensation in the throat
- Tightness or discomfort in the throat or neck location
- Problem swallowing
- Headache
- Trouble breathing (frequently an experience of problem capturing your breath)
- Hardly ever, indigestion or burping might take place
- When the shows are initially begun

Side results might take place. The sensations normally disappear in a couple of hours or days as the individual gets utilized to the settings.

When the settings are increased, they might come back once again momentarily.

If negative effects occur, inform the physician or nurse programs the gadget. Settings can be changed, so the signs do not trouble you.

In many people, negative effects disappear with time.

If negative effects obstruct of particular activities, the stimulation can be shut off momentarily by taping the magnet over the generator.

After the activity is done, get rid of the stimulation, and the magnet will return to its typical pattern.

Examples of when this is done might consist of:

- Hoarseness or cough obstructing of singing or public speaking
- When working out, - Problem capturing your breath.

Does the VNS gadget ever require to be gotten rid of or changed?

- The generator has a battery inside that generally lasts a variety of years.
- When the battery uses down, the generator will require to be changed throughout a brand-new treatment.
- In general, battery shift care takes less than an hour. The person usually goes home the same day.
- After changing a generator, speak with your epilepsy group about when it will be set. You might require to be seen more regularly for a couple of weeks or month up until settings are back to typical for you.
- If an individual feels VNS does not work all right for them, they can have the settings shut off. The gadget does not require to be eliminated.

If required, the generator can be completely eliminated; however, the full lead can not be removed in some situations.

MRI (Magnetic Resonance Imaging).

- Individuals with a VNS gadget can have an MRI; however, specific preventative measures require to be taken.
- Depending upon the VNS gadget implanted, you might require to utilize a unique MRI device. Speak with your epilepsy group prior to scheduling an MRI and ensure the correct device and kind of MRI are reserved.
- The VNS ought to be shut off prior to the MRI. Make a visit with your epilepsy group to have this done prior to going to the MRI space.
- After the MRI, the VNS can be turned back on.

Other Treatments

Individuals who require other treatments or other kinds of surgical treatment might require to follow unique safety measures.

Ask your epilepsy group to inspect and make certain of any security issues for other medical tests or surgical treatments.

Depending on the place on your body or type of surgical treatment or test, you might require to have the VNS turned off. Make certain you established visits with your epilepsy group to do this.

POSSIBLY PREDICTION AND MODULATION OF NON-COMMUNICABLE CHRONIC DISEASES BY VAGUS NERVE

Worldwide disease concern includes non-communicable conditions such as cardiovascular disease, cancer, and persistent obstructive lung disease. Vagal nerve activity is associated with frontal brain activity that controls unhealthy lifestyles.

High vagal disease, measured by increased cardiac disturbances (HRV), epidemiologically, separately predicts decreased GBD hazard and much improved GBD diagnosis. Biological tension, swelling, and considerable activity (and associated hypoxia) of the vagus nerve.

Evaluating the Concern

Significant non-communicable causes of death and of years of life lost today consist of coronary heart problems (CHD), stroke, cancer, and lung illness. Lots of threat aspects (contamination, cigarette smoking, diet-driven cholesterol, inadequate workout, and so on) discuss a big percentage of the significant worldwide problem of illness-- GBD (e.g.,). Numerous of this illness have typical underlying biological causes, as we will see listed below.

Worrying ischemic heart illness (IHD), while rates of myocardial infarction and angina pectoris have actually reduced from 1990 to 2010, the disability-adjusted life years (IHD-burden) increased by 29% in that duration. Significantly, while there is a worldwide reduction in disability-adjusted life years (DALY) from contagious, maternal, nutrition-related, and neonatal illness, there has actually been a boost in DALY from non-communicable illness in between 1990 and 2016. Another pattern is the anticipated increasing concern from persistent obstructive lung illness (COPD) due to increasing contamination in some world areas and due to the aging population.

Intending to battle these patterns, is there one durability element that is epidemiologically associated with significant causes of death, which is associated with behavioral threat aspects contributing to this illness, and which is associated with their typical underlying pathophysiological causes? The prospective modulatory function of the vagus nerve has actually been formerly related to some persistent illness. We then bring clinical proof for the association between these causes of significant illness and vagal nerve activity and epidemiological proof revealing that greater vagal activity forecasts lowered danger of significant persistent illness.

Oxidative Tension and Persistent Illness

Pollution-induced oxidative tension is connected to cardiovascular illness and heart death. Task tension is also associated with higher oxidation (hydrogen peroxide) when looking at mental tension. Persistent stress is observed to be related to the minimum duration of telomeres that forecast illness and premature death.

Swelling and Persistent Illness

Swelling shows the recruitment of immune cells (primarily natural) due to numerous risk signals (e.g., injury, infection, cell damage). Swelling adds to all phases of carcinogenesis from escape from apoptosis and growth, beginning to angiogenesis and transition. Swelling adds to numerous phases of atherogenesis by means of plaque development by macrophage recruitment to severe coronary syndrome by means of producing plaque instability by macrophages, plaque rupture, and superimposed apoplexy.

Psychosocial tension is related to raised pro-inflammatory cytokines and to lowered anti-inflammatory cytokines, in susceptible people. Hence, swelling, the over-reaction of the immune system to threat signals, underlies numerous non-communicable persistent illness.

Extreme Considerate Nerve System Activity and Persistent Illness

Extreme supportive anxious system (SNS) activity is related to cardiovascular illness by causing higher oxygen need from the heart and by causing vasoconstriction, which can cause anemia. Task tension is associated with greater SNS activity. Globalization and increases in financial competitors might result in future greater task tension, decreased work security, and consequently, in more burnout.

Presenting Neuro-Immunology and Neuro-Modulation to Public Health

Medical practice typically looks for to deal with each trigger or contributing aspect of illness independently, by the finest readily available technique. Medically and financially, discovering one element which can prevent all 3 abovementioned aspects at as soon as (oxidative tension, swelling, and considerate hyperactivity), would be far more effective, and might result in fewer side impacts than by 3 different medications. If such a preventing aspect would be discovered, determining its activity must likewise forecast lowered illness threat.

The vagus nerve is the 10th cranial nerve, coming down from the brain stem and getting here to a lot of visceral organs. The vagus nerve is a significant branch of the parasympathetic anxious system, amongst other worried such as the glossopharyngeal and facial nerves. Vagal nerve activity is non-invasively indexed by heart-rate irregularity (HRV), the changes in regular R-R heartbeat periods.

In individuals exposed to tension, just in those with high HRV, brain activity was discovered to be integrated and was associated with peripheral immune and hormone tension actions. This shows the function of the vagus in bridging and in integrating brain and peripheral systems, the secret for neuro-modulation. Notably, vagal nerve activity forecasts the threat of and diagnosis in lots of significant GBD, as we now will see.

Epidemiological Course: Vagal Nerve Activity Anticipates Threat and diagnosis of Persistent Illness

Epidemiological proof reveals inverted associations between vagal nerve activity, indexed by HRV, and the complete metabolic syndrome as well as with the number of its parts. A meta-analysis of 21 research studies discovered that myocardial infarction clients with the SDNN HRV index listed below 70 ms, later on, had around 4 times the threat of death, compared to those with SDNN > 70 ms.

A more recent meta-analysis current that reveals HRV greater predicts considerably anticipates in cancer, and such an association was found to discovered statistically mediated by moderated inflammation Decreased swelling is particular cancer. Therefore, HRV, the vagal nerve index, might be utilized to anticipate the beginning and diagnosis of significant worldwide illness problems.

Biological Course: The Vagus Nerve Hinders Oxidative Tension, Swelling, and Supportive Activity

Empirical proof exists to support the contention that the vagus nerve prevents all 3 significant disease-promoting biological elements discussed above. Vagus nerve stimulation (VNS) decreases oxidative tension. More just recently, scientists discovered in mice with myocardial infarction (MI), that VNS decreased protein oxidation.

These T-cells then produce the vagal neurotransmitter acetylcholine, which binds to the alpha-7 nicotinic acetylcholine receptor on monocyte, resulting in the inhibition of synthesis of inflammatory cytokines. Third, the activity of the vagus nerve, being a significant part of the parasympathetic nerve system, hinders considerate activity.

This is done particularly by vagal nerve caused boosts in vasoactive digestive peptide, which then increases coronary blood circulation. Therefore, biologically, the vagus nerve hinders all 3 promoters of the significant persistent illness pointed out above, and empirical proof supports this.

Behavioral Course: Results of Vagal Activity on Way Of Life Threat Aspects of Persistent Illness

Vagal nerve activity is associated with these ways of life danger elements in a bi-directional way. HRV was substantially lower in cigarette smokers than nonsmokers, and HRV reduced after cigarette smoking amongst cigarette smokers. Notably, vagus nerve activity, indexed by HRV, is favorably associated with executive performance.

Therefore, possibly, by increasing vagus nerve activity, behavioral danger aspects of illness might be decreased as well, through increased executive working. Transcutaneous vagus nerve stimulation (tVNS) led to lowered activity in limbic brain areas, and just recently, likewise to boosts in the anterior cingulate and the left prefrontal cortex.

Vagal nerve stimulation led overweight rats to take in less food, and consequently, to lose weight. One research study discovered that individuals who were high on food yearning, those carrying out HRV-biofeedback, a technique of self-activating one's vagal nerve (through HRV), consequently reported decreases in food yearning compared to controls. As discussed above, it is essential to keep in mind that some of these associations are bi-directional-- for example, physical activity increases HRV.

Ramifications for Avoidance and Treatment: Triggering the Vagal Nerve for Health

Numerous non-pharmacological approaches exist for triggering the vagus nerve. Electrical intrusive and now likewise transcutaneous and non-invasive vagus nerve stimulation (nVNS) gadgets have actually been established. The 2nd non-invasive way is a self-activating type attained by carrying outpaced vagal breathing while getting feedback on one's HRV, called HRV-biofeedback (HRV-B).

One research study discovered HRV-B to cause modifications in swelling in hypertensive clients as a function of modification in HRV. Different kinds of meditation and yoga likewise increase HRV.

There are a number of good medicinal manners to trigger the vagal nerve. However, we will focus on one. It was discovered to increase the level of sensitivity of microalga to radiotherapy in an animal design of glioblastoma.

One just a recently established approach for triggering the vagus electrically is intravenous VNS (iVNS), which was just recently discovered to decrease infarct size in an animal design of myocardial infarction. This might have extensive ramifications for diabetes, a danger element of numerous of the GBD pointed out here. In the coming years, research studies require to check the impacts of such vagal nerve triggering interventions on the persistent illness discussed above, utilizing RCTs.

Keep in mind of Care

Regardless of the epidemiological, biological, and behavioral proof for the reasoning to keep an eye on and potentially trigger the vagal nerve in numerous persistent illnesses, some contrary proof exists. In cancer, non-neuronal autocrine/paracrine acetylcholine, the significant vagal nerve neurotransmitter, might, in reality, potentiate cell development, since preventing its precursor by Bromoachetylcholine bromine, decreased colon cancer cell expansion. Therefore, the distinctions between regional and systemic results of the vagal nerve neurotransmitter need additional examination, and the activation of this nerve requires to be done within a security variety.

From a methodological point of view, concerns of 3rd variables require to be thought about completely when carrying out longitudinal observational or interventional RCT, to separate the assumed contribution of the vagus nerve in avoiding GBD. If vagal nerve activation will be evaluated and utilized in the future to potentially avoid and deal with particular GBD, problems of frequency, period, and strength of vagal activation requirement to be checked per illness, while constantly thinking about security concerns.

Persistent non-communicable illnesses can be deadly; they are widespread and present a substantial person, social, financial, and medical concern. The vagus nerve decreases specific behavioral threat aspects and prevents 3 primary pathophysiological elements that contribute to that illness (oxidative tension, swelling, and extreme SNS activity).

At the epidemiological level, HRV, the vagal nerve index, anticipates the danger of this illness, and numerous research studies reveal helpful results of vagal nerve activation on the pathophysiological factors, on the behavioral threat elements and on some of this deadly illness. Future research studies must check-in massive trials the impacts of vagal nerve activation on this illness, to minimize the worldwide problem resulting from them.

PHARMACOLOGICAL MODULATION OF VAGAL NERVE ACTIVITY IN CARDIOVASCULAR DISEASES

Presently, medicinal interventions mostly intend to hinder over-excitation of considerate nerves, while vagal modulation has actually been mainly ignored. Lots of research studies have actually shown that increased vagal activity minimizes cardiovascular danger aspects in both animal designs and human clients. The enhancement of vagal activity might be an alternate technique for the treatment of cardiovascular illness.

ANS imbalances that are found in the vagal tone, together with increasing significant activity, are associated with the production of disease and adverse medical effects that can lead to loads of cardiovascular diseases including cardiac arrhythmias, inadequate breathing, and high blood pressure. However, various research findings have shown that increased vagus activity decreases cardiovascular-hazard factors both in animal and human projects. Medications that activate vagal nerves and vagomimetic medications in the treatment of cardiovascular disease are not yet fully understood.

In today's evaluation, we sum up the current research studies detailing the substance abuse in vagal nerve activation for the treatment of heart disease, in addition to putative systems underlying the cardiovascular protective results of these substances.

Modification of Vagal Tone in Heart Disease

The heart system is controlled by both strongly and parasympathetic nerves. Vagal and protective muscles complement the innervation unbalanced. Ideal intelligence and vagal nerves that encircle the sinus node and atrium primarily regulate cardiac contractility and heart production, and the left comprehension and vagal nerves that encircle the left ventricle and auriculo-ventricular interface.

Under physiological conditions, the parasympathetic and considerate (vagal) activities regulating heart function go through a mutual guideline, leading to sympathovagal balance. All at once, the vagal nerve releases ACh to decrease the conduction of pacemaker cells in the sinus node, therefore decreasing the heart rate and the myocardial contractility.

Reduced vagal nerve discharge and a reduction in the quantity of ACh launched into the synaptic cleft, leading to the loss of the capability of the vagal nerve to minimize the heart rate and reduce myocardial contractility. Hence, the repair or improvement of vagal nerve activity might be an appealing treatment for cardiovascular illness.

The activation of vagal nerves takes place at numerous levels, consisting of the afferent, main, and efferent parts and all associated effectors. Our main issue is the relationship between activation of the vagal efferent element and heart disease. Vagal afferents can be triggered throughout the following procedures: a boost in neuronal discharge and ACh release by activation of the main axis and direct vagal nerve stimulation; the administration of cholinergic drugs or the indirect boost in ACh levels by administration of cholinesterase inhibitors; and a boost in ACh bioavailability by activation of the ACh-associated receptors (M receptors and the N receptor) and downstream paths.

BRS is mostly related to as a step of a vagal reflex activity and is revealed in milliseconds of the boost in the RR period ensuing a boost of 1 mmHg in blood pressure. Other techniques, such as the ACh level in the blood determined by microdialysis, heart automated nerves and cholinergic nerve circulation by immunohistochemistry, free tone and intrinsic heart rate by administration of atropine and propranolol or neuronal/vagal discharge determined by a biological signal analytical system, can likewise be utilized to assess vagal activity in experiments.

Reduced Vagal Tone is Connected With Increased Death in Cardiac Arrest

It has actually been shown that reduced vagal tone is associated with a boost in death for HF. Reduced ventricular epicardial vagal nerve density has actually likewise been reported to possibly contribute to impaired heart vagal control in rats with HF. For the treatment of HF, vagus nerve stimulation (VNS) has actually been revealed to be advantageous for enhancing the free balance in HF by boosting vagal tone.

Arrhythmia with Decreased Vagal Tone after Myocardial Infarction

Arrhythmia is a deadly threat of reduced vagal tone accompanying myocardial infarction. We actually reported that cholinergic nerves and M2 receptors are both the rat atrium and the ventricle. Initiating and enhancing vagal control of arhythmia plays an important role, and the recent invention of vagomimetic medication will hold treatment secrets.

Minimized Vagal Activity Adds To Hypertensive Organ Damage

Vagal nerve fibers can regulate systemic and regional inflammatory reactions, understood as the 'cholinergic anti-inflammatory path.' Our group likewise showed that a boost in the expression of TLR4 and pro-inflammatory cytokines might be associated with reduced vagal activity in SHRs. The increasing vagal activity might be an intriguing alternative technique for antihypertensive treatment.

Unusual ANS activity is associated with lots of other heart diseases, such as myocardial infarction, ischemia/reperfusion injury, and atherosclerosis. In summary, the vagal nerve plays a crucial function in lots of heart diseases, and even more, the examination is needed to discover treatments for bringing back impaired vagal nerve function to enhance medical results and diagnoses.

POSSIBLE TARGETS FOR VAGAL NERVE ACTIVATION IN HEART DISEASE

Muscarinic Receptors and Cardiovascular Diseases

Cholinergic receptors are traditionally divided into 2 types of ACh receptors (AChRs), particularly, the nicotinic and muscarinic receptors.

The muscarinic ACh receptor (mAChR) is a member of a sub-family of G protein-coupled receptors that consists of the M1-- M5 subtypes.

Our research studies have actually likewise revealed that ACh hinders growth necrosis element alpha production by downregulating p38 mitogen-activated protein kinase (MAPK) and JNK phosphorylation; this is moderated by the M2 receptor, and M2 villains or the knockdown of M2 receptor expression by siRNA eliminates the results of ACh-induced defense in cardiomyocytes. Current research studies have actually discovered that the M3 receptor subtype is likewise dispersed in myocardial cells, and plays a protective function in heart disease.

Some research studies have actually reported that M3 receptor activation decreases angiotensin II-induced heart hypertrophy, fixes hemodynamic heart dysfunction, prevents myocardial cell apoptosis, and lowers myocardial injury. A cardioprotective effect of the medicinal activation of M3 receptors is also an is chemically caused by ischemia / reperfusion (I / R) injury.

Nicotinic Acetylcholine Receptors and Cardiovascular Diseases

The nicotinic ACh receptors (nAchRs) consist of 5 ion channels which delimit a principal liquid pore. The ACh binds to α7nAchR, which prevents p38 MAPK and nuclear factor-Kappa B transcription activity. In addition, Janus kinase 2 (Jak2) may also be hired by α7nAchR to create an intracellular transductive action moderated by transcription signal transducer / activator 3 (STAT3).

Vagal stimulation safeguards versus myocardial I/R-induced remote vascular dysfunction through the cholinergic anti-inflammatory path, which depends on α7nACh receptors. Previous research studies have actually likewise revealed that α7nACh receptors obstruct inflammasome complex activation by reducing mitochondrial DNA release. The medicinal activation of α7nAchR, Defines an alternative cardiovascular disease management technique by enhancing vagal activity.

β2 Adrenergic Receptors and Heart Disease

Adrenergic receptors (ARs) are a big household of seven-transmembrane domain receptors responsive to catecholamines. These research studies have actually shown that β2AR-activated T cells in the spleen are crucial for the anti-inflammatory action of the vagus nerve, and β2ARs represent a prospective medicinal target for vagal activation in cardiovascular illness.

Drugs for Cardioprotection by Vagal Nerve Activation

Modulation of the vagal nerve activity is, in theory, an appealing treatment for cardiovascular illness. Present, significant, non-drug-activated vagal nerve activation methods consist of direct vagal stimulation through surgically implanted stimulators, and indirect kidney sympathectomy, aerobic workout, and yoga.

There is currently much proof that direct VNS can efficiently enhance the event and advancement of cardiovascular illness, due to surgical injury, bad client compliance, and an insufficient reaction in clients with heart deficiency, its prevalent application in the center has actually been restricted. The vagus nerve stimulation by means of medication could be another way to control VNS for customers with cardiovascular disease. Vagomimetic medications that enhance the nicotine and muscarinic receptor levels of synaptic ACh are the main targets used in cardiac nerve activation; cholinesterase indirectly decreases the degradation of ACh;

and adenosine, statins, beta-receptor blockers, and angiotensin-converting-enzyme inhibitors (ACEIs), which likewise indirectly trigger vagal tone; nevertheless, the hidden systems through which these drugs promote vagal activation still need additional examination.

CHOLINERGIC SUBSTANCE ABUSE IN THE TREATMENT OF HEART DISEASE

Choline

Collecting proof has actually shown that choline likewise has several protective results versus numerous cardiovascular illness, consisting of myocardial infarction, arrhythmias, heart hypertrophy, and I/R injury. Choline has actually likewise been shown to have a protective impact versus vascular damage in rats after I/R through the inhibition of the reactive oxygen types (ROS)-moderated Ca2+/ calmodulin-dependent protein kinase II (CaMKII) path and the guideline of Ca2+biking proteins.

These protective impacts might be associated with the activation of the M3 receptor. These protective results might be related to the enhancement in vagal activity and the decrease in inflammatory cytokines discovered in SHRs.

Acetylcholine

ACh has two main types of cholinoceptor, and it is probably a unique drug development goal, nicotine and musculoskeletal agonist. Work in vitro microdialysis has shown that vagal stimulation raises ACh production in the mesenteric bloodstream, indicates migration of ACh from the vagus nerve into mesenteric circulation and results in endothelial and vascular smooth cells. In this study, studies have been conducted. Research studies in our lab have actually shown that ACh avoids angiotensin II-induced cardiomyocyte injury through down-regulation of the angiotensin II type 1 receptor and inhibition of ROS-mediated p38 MAPK activation, along with the policy of Caspase-3, Bax, and BCL-2 expression.

Our research studies suggested that ACh attenuates intracellular Ca2+ overload by hindering the development of the VDAC1/Grp75/IP3R1 complex and the NCX1-TRPC3-IP3R1 complex in mitochondria-endoplasmic reticulum and endoplasmic reticulum-plasma membrane connection websites in human umbilical vein endothelial cells, showing that the inhibition of inter-organelle crosstalk might be a system for vagal protective results in cardiovascular illness. Presently, ACh is mainly utilized as a pharmaceutical tool due to the several impacts that it has throughout the body.

ACETYLCHOLINESTERASE INHIBITORS FOR THE TREATMENT OF HEART DISEASE

Pyridostigmine

In addition, the advancement of brand-new shipment approaches (e.g., nanoparticles and liposomes) might lower the side-effects of PYR. Proof has actually revealed that long-lasting treatment with PYR increases heart vagal tone, decreases considerate tone, and attenuates heart renovation and left ventricular dysfunction throughout the development of HF in mice.

More current research studies have actually shown essential functions for PYR in maintaining free balance. The most current research study likewise showed that the administration of PYR for 12 weeks ameliorates the cardiomyopathy caused by a high-fat diet plan in Sprague-Dawley rats, which is accompanied by enhanced vagal activity, minimized heart lipid build-up, and the assisted in browning of white adipose tissue while triggering brown adipose tissue. Research studies are still essential to much better comprehend the pleiotropic results of PYR on cardiovascular security.

OTHER DRUGS FOR CARDIOVASCULAR SECURITY (ADENOSINE, STATINS, B-RECEPTOR BLOCKERS, AND ACEIS).

Adenosine

Our research study likewise showed a possible practical interaction between muscarinic M2 receptors and $\alpha1$ adenosine receptors in the I/R myocardium, and nitric oxide synthase might be the link between these 2 types of receptors. The precursor of adenosine (adenine sulfate) has actually likewise been recommended to have cardioprotective impacts by increasing the expression of M2 receptors and cholinergic nerve density. A current research study recommended that the repressive impacts of VNS on HR and BP are partially moderated by endogenous adenosine release.

Statins

Our previous research study showed that atorvastatin improves serum ACh levels and baroreflex levels of sensitivity in I/R injury in rats. In a human research study, atorvastatin likewise had a helpful effect on vagal activity, as determined by enhancements in HRV, and may lower the danger for arrhythmias in HF clients. A current research study recommended that statins may enhance and lower arrhythmias HRV in healthy individuals after 48 h of sleep deprivation.

β-Adrenoceptor Blockers

Their protective impact is not totally reliant on the direct blockade of understanding activity. The afferent understanding excitation results in the activation of considerate efferent activity, together with the inhibition of vagal activity. The cardiovascular protective impacts applied by β-blockers are due mostly to inhibition of the β1 receptor.

A previous research study revealed that carvedilol (an α- and β-blocker) increases the expression of M2 receptors in myocardium hurt by adriamycin, suggesting that the up-regulation of these muscarinic receptors might be instrumental for the protective impacts of carvedilol in HF. It has actually likewise been reported that long-lasting treatment with carvedilol brings back free tone and responsiveness in clients with moderate HF. Vagal activation caused by metoprolol, another β-blocker, avoids ventricular fibrillation in mice with dilated cardiomyopathy.

Angiotensin-Converting-Enzyme Inhibitors

A current study has also shown that enalapril increases its vagal tone with aerobic physical training. ACEI may be an enticing vagomimetic cardiovascular drug, but further research studies are required in order to understand the mechanism.

VAGUS NERVE STIMULATION

Vagus nerve stimulation includes making use of a gadget to promote the vagus nerve with electrical impulses. An implantable vagus nerve stimulator is presently FDA-approved to deal with epilepsy and anxiety. There's one vagus nerve on each side of your body, ranging from your brainstem through your neck to your chest and abdominal area.

In standard vagus nerve stimulation, a gadget is surgically implanted under the skin on your chest, and a wire is threaded under your skin linking the gadget to the left vagus nerve. When triggered, the gadget sends out electrical signals along the left vagus nerve to your brainstem, which then sends out signals to particular locations in your brain. Due to the fact that it's more most likely to bring fibers that provide nerves to the heart, the best vagus nerve isn't utilized.

New, noninvasive vagus nerve stimulation gadgets, which do not need surgical implantation, have actually been authorized in Europe to deal with discomfort, epilepsy, and anxiety. A noninvasive gadget that promotes the vagus nerve was just recently authorized by the Fda for the treatment of cluster headaches in the United States.

Why it's done

About one-third of individuals with epilepsy do not completely react to anti-seizure drugs. Vagus nerve stimulation might be an alternative to minimize the frequency of seizures in individuals who have not attained control with medications.

Vagus nerve stimulation might likewise be handy for individuals who have not reacted to extensive anxiety treatments, such as antidepressant medications, mental therapy (psychiatric therapy), and electroconvulsive treatment (ECT).

The Fda (FDA) has actually authorized vagus nerve stimulation for individuals who:

- Are 4 years of ages and older
- Have focal (partial) epilepsy
- Have seizures that aren't well-controlled with medications

The FDA has actually likewise authorized vagus nerve stimulation for the treatment of anxiety in grownups who:

- Have persistent, hard-to-treat anxiety (treatment-resistant anxiety)
- Have not enhanced after attempting 4 or more medications or electroconvulsive treatment (ECT), or both
- Continue basic anxiety treatments together with vagus nerve stimulation

Furthermore, scientists are studying vagus nerve stimulation as a prospective treatment for a range of conditions, consisting of headaches, rheumatoid arthritis, inflammatory bowel illness, bipolar illness, weight problems, and Alzheimer's illness.

Threats

For many people, vagus nerve stimulation is safe. It does have some dangers, both from the surgical treatment to implant the gadget and from the brain stimulation.

Surgical treatment dangers

Surgical problems with implanted vagus nerve stimulation are unusual and resemble the risks of having other kinds of surgical treatment.

They consist of:

- Discomfort where the cut (cut) is made to implant the gadget
- Infection
- Problem swallowing
- Singing cable paralysis, which is normally short-lived, however, can be irreversible

Adverse effects after surgical treatment

A few of the negative effects and illnesses connected with implanted vagus nerve stimulation can consist of:

- Voice modifications
- Hoarseness
- Throat discomfort
- Cough
- Headaches
- Shortness of breath
- Problem swallowing
- Tingling or tingling of the skin

- Sleeping disorders
- Worsening of sleep apnea

For the majority of people, adverse effects are bearable. They might decrease with time. However, some adverse effects might stay annoying for as long as you utilize implanted vagus nerve stimulation.

Changing the electrical impulses can assist decrease these results. The gadget can be shut off briefly or completely if side impacts are excruciating.

How you prepare

It is essential to thoroughly think about the benefits and drawbacks of implanted vagus nerve stimulation prior to choosing to have the treatment. Ensure you understand what all of your other treatment options are, which you and your physician both feel that implanted vagus nerve stimulation is the very best alternative for you. Ask your physician precisely what you need to anticipate throughout surgical treatment and after the pulse generator remains in location.

Food and medications

You might require to stop taking particular medications ahead of time, and your medical professional might ask you not to consume the night prior to the treatment.

WHAT YOU CAN ANTICIPATE

Prior to the treatment

Prior to surgical treatment, your physician will do a health examination. You might require blood tests or other tests to ensure you do not have any health issues that may be an issue. Your physician might have you begin taking prescription antibiotics prior to surgical treatment to avoid infection.

Throughout the treatment

Surgical treatment to implant the vagus nerve stimulation gadget can be done on an outpatient basis, though some cosmetic surgeons advise remaining overnight.

The surgical treatment normally takes an hour to a half and an hour. You might stay awake; however, have medication to numb the surgical treatment location (regional anesthesia), or you might be unconscious throughout the surgical treatment (basic anesthesia).

The surgical treatment itself does not include your brain. 2 cuts are made, one on your chest or in the underarm (axillary) area, and the other on the left side of the neck.

The pulse generator is implanted in the upper left side of your chest. The gadget is suggested to be a long-term implant. However, it can be gotten rid of if required.

The pulse generator has to do with the size of a stop-watch and operates on battery power. A lead wire is linked to the pulse generator. The lead wire is directed under your skin from your chest approximately your neck, where it's connected to the left vagus nerve through the 2nd cut.

After the treatment

The pulse generator is switched on throughout a see to your physician's workplace a couple of weeks after surgical treatment. It can be set to provide electrical impulses to the vagus nerve at different periods, currents, and frequencies. Vagus nerve stimulation normally begins at a low level and is slowly increased, depending upon your signs and negative effects.

Stimulation is set to switch on and off in particular cycles-- such as 30 seconds on, 5 minutes off. When the nerve stimulation is on, you might have some tingling feelings or small discomfort in your neck and momentary hoarseness.

The stimulator does not spot seizure activity or anxiety signs. The stimulator turns on and off at the periods chosen by your medical professional when it's turned on. You can utilize a hand-held magnet to start stimulation at various times, for instance, if you notice an approaching seizure.

The magnet can likewise be utilized to momentarily shut off the vagus nerve stimulation, which might be needed when you do specific activities such as public speaking, singing, or working out, or when you're consuming if you have swallowing issues.

You'll require to visit your physician regularly to ensure that the pulse generator is working properly, which it hasn't moved out of position. Consult your physician prior to having any medical tests, such as magnetic resonance imaging (MRI), which may hinder your gadget.

Outcomes

Implanted vagus nerve stimulation isn't a treatment for epilepsy. A lot of individuals with epilepsy will not stop taking or having seizures epilepsy medication entirely after the treatment.

It can take months or perhaps a year or longer of stimulation prior to you observe any considerable decrease in seizures. Vagus nerve stimulation might likewise reduce the healing time after a seizure. Individuals who have actually had vagus nerve stimulation to deal with epilepsy might likewise experience enhancements in state of mind and lifestyle.

The research study is still blended on the advantages of implanted vagus nerve stimulation for the treatment of anxiety. Some research studies recommend the advantages of vagus nerve stimulation for anxiety accumulate gradually, and it might take a minimum of a number of months of treatment prior to you discover any enhancements in your anxiety signs. Implanted vagus nerve stimulation does not work for everyone, and it isn't meant to change standard treatments.

Furthermore, some medical insurance providers might not spend on this treatment.

Research studies of implanted vagus nerve stimulation as a treatment for conditions such as Alzheimer's illness, headaches, and rheumatoid arthritis have actually been too little to draw any conclusive conclusions about how well it might work for those issues.

HOW TO ACTIVATE THE VAGUS NERVE ON YOUR OWN?

Vagus nerve stimulation can be switched on quickly though a variety of breathing and relaxation strategies:

- Deep/slow tummy breathing
- ' OM' Shouting
- Coldwater face immersion after a workout
- Filling the mouth with saliva and immersing your tongue to activate a hyper-relaxing vagal
- action.
- Loud swishing with water
- Loud singing

To practice deep breathing, breathe in through your nose and breathe out through your mouth.

Keep in mind to:

- Breathe more gradually.
- Breathe more deeply, from the stomach.
- Exhale longer than you breathe in.

Utilizing Breathing to Lower Discomfort

If you focus on the rhythm of your breathing, you're not focused on the discomfort. The minute we expect discomfort, many of us tend to stop breathing and hold our breath.

Breath-holding triggers the fight/flight/freeze action; it tends to increase the feeling of discomfort, stress and anxiety, tightness, or worry.

You should go on like this: Take a deep inhalation into your belly (i.e., expand your diaphragm) at 5, spawn, and then gradually breathe out through a small hole in your mouth. Breathing out through your mouth rather than your nose makes breathing more thoughtful and helps you observe your breathing faster.

As you decrease your breaths per minute and get into parasympathetic mode, your muscles will unwind, dropping your stress and anxieties, and concerns. Tibetan monks have actually been practicing 'mindful breathing' for years. However, there is absolutely nothing strange about it.

' OM' Shouting

The 2011 International Journal of Yoga published an interesting research project, where' OM ' screams relative to' SSS' pronunciation and a rest state were matched to figure out if chanting was more relaxing for the slightly tense. The study found that screaming was, in fact, more confident than the pronunciation "sss" or the remainder.

Efficient 'OM' shouting is connected with the experience of a vibration feeling around the ears and throughout the body. It is anticipated that such a feeling is likewise sent through the auricular branch of the vagus nerve and will produce limbic (HPA axis) deactivation.fiii]

How to shout?

Hold the vowel (o) part of the 'OM' for 5 seconds then continue into the consonant (m) part for the next 10 seconds. Continue chanting for 10 minutes. Conclude with some deep breathing and end with appreciation.

Cold Water

Physical workout triggers a boost in supportive activity (HPA axis - fight/flight, tension action), along with parasympathetic withdrawal (resting, absorbing, recovery, immune system), resulting in greater heart rates (HR). Research studies have actually discovered that cold water face immersion appears to be an effective and basic method of instantly speeding up post-exercise parasympathetic reactivation through the vagus nerve, promoting the decrease of heart rate, motility of the intestinal tracts, and turns on the immune system. It is likewise efficient in a non-exercise environment to trigger the vagus nerve.

The calmer the mind and the much deeper the relaxation, the simpler the stimulation of salivation is. When the mouth is able to produce generous quantities of saliva, you understand that the Vagus Nerve has actually been promoted, and your body is in the parasympathetic mode. As your mouth fills with saliva, simply rest your tongue in this bath (if this does not take place, simply fill your mouth with a little quantity of warm water and rest your tongue in this bath.

EXISTS A FUNCTION FOR VAGUS NERVE STIMULATION IN THE TREATMENT OF POSTTRAUMATIC TENSION CONDITION?

Posttraumatic tension condition (PTSD) establishes in people who have actually been exposed to injury and subsequently suffer distress or practical disability for at least 1 month. Current natural catastrophes, mass shootings, terrorist attacks, and cities under siege include the international concern of PTSD, which, according to a 2017 research study, impacts 4-- 6% of the worldwide population, although the bulk of injuries are associated to mishaps and physical or sexual violence.

A PTSD psychopharmacology working group just recently released their agreement declaration calling for instant action to deal with the crisis in PTSD treatment, mentioning 3 significant issues. Just 2 drugs (sertraline and paroxetine) are authorized by the United States FDA for the treatment of PTSD. PTSD clients are recommended medications to attend to each of their numerous special and varied signs consisting of stress and anxiety, trouble sleeping, sexual dysfunction, anxiety, and persistent discomfort, with inadequate empirical examinations of drug interactions.

Direct exposure treatment depends on the procedure of snuffing out the conditioned worry memory, which is gotten rid of by a brand-new memory that establishes through duplicated direct exposures. The clients with stress and anxiety conditions and PTSD reveal problems in their capability to snuff out conditioned worries, which might contribute to the advancement of conditions and might interfere with development in treatment.

Due to the fact that the memory of the injury is not lost, however, rather, enhancements through treatment depend upon brand-new found out associations that take on distressing associations; the balance of the 2 memories can move with time, causing regression. Other obstacles consist of the trouble in snuffing out and acknowledging worry of all conditioned stimuli, and a high dropout rate, which is not unexpected, considered that avoidance is among the signs of PTSD.

Outcomes of research studies evaluating the results of cognitive enhancers as accessories to direct exposure treatment are blended in the case of PTSD. A possible description is that drugs offered prior to direct exposure treatment sessions run the danger of enhancing unfavorable associations if direct exposure produces stress and anxiety.

Results suggest that anxiolytic drugs do not improve the results of direct exposure treatment. One description is that the stress and anxiety action is needed for success in direct exposure treatment due to the fact that clients should discover not to fear their own worry action. A perfect accessory would tap into the systems that improve the combination of distressing memories in order to promote termination memories that are simply as strong, all the while bypassing or preventing the aversive tension action.

Emerging proof recommends that vagus nerve stimulation (VNS) might be an advantageous accessory to exposure-based treatments through its pairing-specific improvement of memory debt consolidation and neural plasticity. It signifies the brain throughout times of increased understanding activity, promoting quick storage of memories that are crucial for survival.

VNS improves memory in people and rats, recommending that combining VNS with unreinforced direct exposure to conditioned hints might improve the combination of the termination memory. Comprehensive proof suggests that VNS promotes neural plasticity, specifically when it is combined with training, and this result includes VNS modulation of the locus coeruleus noradrenergic system.

VNS-treated rats likewise carried out much better on tests of stress and anxiety, stimulation, avoidance, and social interactions 1 week, later on, showing that turnaround of the termination disability equated to enhancements in other PTSD signs. In addition, persistent, unpaired VNS, as is utilized in the treatment of epilepsy and anxiety, enhanced efficiency on the Hamilton Stress And Anxiety Scale in some clients with stress and anxiety conditions, and lowered anxiety-like habits in rats.

The impacts of VNS on termination in our research studies are not seen when the VNS is administered 30 minutes to 1 h after training. These findings recommend that VNS might decrease stress and anxiety; however, pairing-specific plasticity and memory modulation is required for termination improvement. Our current, unpublished findings suggest that rats are more most likely to check out the open arms of a raised plus labyrinth instantly after getting VNS, recommending that VNS produces a severe anxiolytic impact.

VNS increases monoamine in the locus, and the brain coeruleus processes as VNS-induced seizures are reduced. The medical practice of VNS involves the operative implantation of an electrode attached by a cut in the neck to the left cervical vacuum nerve.

Surgical problems, such as infection or singing cable results, happen in about 1% of clients. These were not regulated research studies, and Corning deserted the method since of side impacts such as lightheadedness and syncope; nevertheless, transcutaneous VNS (t-VNS) has actually just recently restored status as a medical tool.

With this t-VNS, the electrical stimulus, with a strength that is above sensory detection, however, listed below the discomfort limit, is used through the skin to the responsive field of the auricular branch. Blended outcomes were seen in a current research study taking a look at t-VNS results on termination of conditioned worry in human beings, and scientific research study on making use of t-VNS is restricted. However, it appears to be safe and well endured. Transcutaneous variations of VNS might offer the advantages of VNS without the threats of surgical treatment; nevertheless, t-VNS is not yet a recognized treatment, and the decision of its effectiveness needs more examination.

VNS holds guarantee as an accessory to exposure-based treatments due to the fact that it improves memory debt consolidation and promotes synaptic plasticity while moistening the understanding tension action. VNS has actually been utilized in people for over 2 years, the practice of matching it with direct exposure treatment has actually not been evaluated in clients, and numerous concerns stay unanswered.

Some proof shows that persistent VNS decreases stress and anxiety in human beings and in rats. If VNS can right away lower stress and anxiety, this may, or might not be useful for exposure-based treatments. Research studies are presently underway to figure out whether various stimulation criteria can be utilized to dissociate memory results of VNS from anxiolytic impacts.

The neural plasticity that underlies terrible memories can be adaptive, decreasing the possibility that unsafe habits will be duplicated. Periodically, terrible memories have maladaptive repercussions, leading to stress and anxiety- or stress-related conditions. We intend to harness the capacity of the vagus nerve to drive neural plasticity throughout direct exposure treatment, while simultaneously disrupting the understanding fight-or-flight reaction.

VAGUS NERVE STIMULATION MAY CONTROL EPILEPSY

One alternative that can be looked after attempting dietary treatment is Vagus Nerve Stimulation. This is a medical gadget that is surgically implanted. Any significant medical center in the United States and Europe can implant this gadget for a client that certifies.

Vagus Nerve Stimulation (VNS) includes sending out a message to the brain utilizing regular moderate electrical stimulation from the vagus nerve in the neck by a surgically implanted little medical gadget. This stimulation or pulse is sent out by a medical gadget comparable to a pacemaker.

VNS might manage epilepsy in cases where anti-epileptic drugs are inadequate or have unbearable negative effects, or neurosurgery is not proper for some factor. VNS works in stopping seizures in some clients.

The implanted medical gadget is a flat, round battery and determines the size of a silver dollar. The VNS medical gadget was established by Cyberonics, Inc.

The side impacts of VNS throughout treatment might consist of hoarseness, coughing, throat discomfort, shortness of breath, a small and brief feeling of choking, transformed voice noise, ear discomfort, tooth discomfort, and a tingling feeling in the neck. For those with unmanageable epileptic seizures, it might be the last choice. Think about all alternatives prior to providing up on managing seizure.

VAGUS NERVE STIMULATION TREATMENT CAN REMOVE DRUG YEARNINGS

Dependency on any compound can make the life of a private topsy-turvy. There are numerous aspects of play when it comes to dealing with the growing issue of dependency.

Yearnings are a severe concern that torture various individuals battling drug dependency, specifically when they attempt to come off the addicting compound. Paradoxically, many individuals would have effectively obtained long-lasting sobriety if yearnings did not emerge with dependency. Apart from being thought about as the significant challenges in healing treatment, yearnings are likewise the origin of regression.

When an individual is totally free from yearnings, total healing from dependency occurs just. Living a drug-free life without the requirement for continuous tracking versus drug yearnings can be tough for a recuperating specific; however, a current research study released in the journal Knowing and Memory has actually recommended that drug yearnings can be successfully treated with vagus nerve stimulation (VNS) treatment. Undertreatment, the clients are taught brand-new habits that change their old addicting habits of looking for drugs.

The function of VNS in dependency healing

In the University of Texas at Dallas research study, the scientists exposed that the VNS treatment assisted clients to recuperate from the maladaptive habits of drug-taking. It mainly works by sending out minor electrical pulses through the vagus nerve, which even more reaches the brain, therefore managing the yearnings and advice.

The method is authorized by the U.S. Food and Drug Administration (FDA) and is thought about as a possible treatment for treatment-resistant anxiety, post-traumatic tension condition (PTSD), and paralysis. The research study, even more, highlighted that VNS helps with "termination knowing" of drug-seeking habits by minimizing yearnings and changing the habits associated with a dependency with brand-new ones.

Drug-free life is possible

Addicting compounds be successful in briefly relieving the physical and psychological discomforts of drug abusers; they have to cope with the agonizing signs of compound abuse ultimately. Establishing a number of psychological and physical issues, numerous of these people likewise end up being self-destructive and self-destructive in nature.

Dependency on any compound can be lethal. The degree to which health care specialists can amass outcomes in the treatment for drug dependency is reliant on the scientific qualities of the clients that might differ according to the type of drug being abused as well as its amount, period and the approach of utilizing the drug (intravenous or oral).

ONE ESSENTIAL THING MEDICAL PROFESSIONALS FORGET TO INFORM YOU ABOUT VNS SURGICAL TREATMENT

Vagus Nerve Stimulation surgical treatment, a desperate effort to manage seizures, stimulate debate among those who have actually the gadget implanted. Lots of clients enjoy the remedy for unmanageable seizures. Numerous other clients dislike the side-effects triggered by surgical treatment and development.

Approximately 70 percent of individuals might have their seizures managed with prescription drugs. For the staying 30 percent, surgical treatment might be an alternative. Epilepsy surgical treatment has several variations; temporal lobe resection, extratemporal cortical resection, and corpus callosal area.

These extreme surgical treatments, Vagus or Vagal Nerve Stimulation surgical treatment (VNS), implants a VNS pulse generator under the skin of the chest in a surgically produced pocket. The VNS utilizes electrical pulses provided to the vagus nerve in the neck, which takes a trip up into the brain.

No one understands why the VNS lowers seizures. Clients report that VNS lowers the number, length, intensity of seizures, and the length of healing time after seizures.

One crucial thing physicians forget to inform you prior to the implant the VNS in a $23,000 surgical treatment: If you have a heart attack, you can not be treated with an automatic external defibrillator (AED). Clients with VNS can not get first aid with electrical charges utilized to bring back regular heart rhythm to clients in a heart attack.

THE VAGUS NERVE, YOUR MEDITATION HIGHWAY, AND THE PARASYMPATHETIC NERVE SYSTEM; HOW MEDITATION WORKS FAVORABLY ON THE BODY

Buddhism is understood for its focus on meditation and meditative strategies. Individuals from all strolls of life have actually utilized Buddhist strategies to 'unwind' and 'de-stress,' regardless of neither being practicing Buddhists nor undoubtedly comprehending much (if anything) about Buddhism itself. Without a doubt, meditation and the meditative methods established by Buddhists have actually assisted a fantastic numerous to manage stress and anxiety and psychological health concerns, without always comprehending their much deeper significance.

Advances in the field of psychiatry, and a stronger desire to correctly examine psychological health concerns has actually brought clinical regard for the recovery capacity of meditation.

They have actually found a lot-- however, one of the most intriguing (and lower understood) findings worries the action of meditative methods upon the vagus nerve.

The Vagus Nerve-- the Meditation Highway?

Put merely; it's one of the longest nerves in your body (a sciatic nerve is the longest). The vagus nerve takes a trip from your brainstem, winding down throughout your body, to complete in your abdominal area. We have actually been conscious of it for a really long time and been likewise conscious of the truth that the vagus nerve is semi-responsible for your body's policy of heart rate, breathing rate, food digestion, and so forth.It was formerly presumed that the vagus nerve acted more or less on its own effort- that is, without the mindful input of the person.

Research study exposed the deeply interconnected method in which awareness and physicality can affect one another-- and the vagus nerve. Explained by some as a 'hack' to the nerve system, the vagus nerve seems science's response to the vexed concern of simply how, specifically, Buddhist practices do what they do. And this type of clinical confirmation and understanding has actually come in the nick of time; a growing number of people, it appears, need the advantages of 'vagal nerve stimulation.'

Modern Mental Dysfunction-- and 'Detached' Individuals

It's an unfortunate reality that psychological health issues associated with tension and stress and anxiety are immensely on the increase. Some professionals think we are normally more mindful of psychological health issues than we utilized to be, and that we're likewise more most likely to look for aid for medical problems in basic.

On a more spiritual level, modern-day (and Western in specific) society has actually been implicated in developing 'detached' individuals, having a hard time to discover a sense of identity, a sense of self, and fundamental spiritual satisfaction in a quickly altering world. Whatever the factor, we're certainly suffering from a surfeit of stress and anxiety-- which can be really hazardous.

Tension and stress and anxiety can trigger any variety of psychological health problems, which can, in turn, cause physical health problems (drug abuse springs right away to mind). We have actually understood for a long time that meditation (or 'mindfulness'-- the nonreligious, clinical, and significantly popular meditative practice) can aid with a number of these issues.

As meditation ends up being more popular, increasingly more individuals wish to dissect the secrets of meditation and get to the bottom of what makes it so efficient. No clinical physician would recommend a treatment-- nevertheless reliable it's been shown to be-- without comprehending it incomplete, analytical information. This is where the vagus nerve can be found in.

The Parasympathetic and considerate Nerve system

One of these is the 'considerate anxious system'-- accountable for the 'Battle or Flight' response. Your understanding of the anxious system is one branch of the 'free worried system'-- so-called due to the fact that it's thought to act 'autonomously' (i.e., automatically). The other primary branch of the free anxious system is the 'parasympathetic anxious system'-- about which we are in basic substantially less notified.

The parasympathetic anxious system is accountable for the so-called 'Rest and Digest' functions, and we do not pay as much attention to it as we should. To cut a long story short, when we practice meditation, we motivate our body to change functional control from the 'Battle or Flight' system to the 'Rest and Digest' system.

External Anxious Stimulation

We all understand slightly how the 'Battle or Flight' response works-- we're frightened by something, and our anxious understanding system jumps into action to offer us the 'increase' we require in order to either battle or leave our method out of threat. The 'Battle or Flight' response can feel thrilling in brief bursts-- it's why we ride rollercoasters-- however, it's not developed to last more than half an hour at the most.

Our 'Battle or Flight' response is created to assist us to leave lions-- however, it's being triggered by the needs of self-important managers. And that's just terrible for our health.

What must take place is that our considerate worried system needs to naturally deliver control to our parasympathetic anxious system once the risk is previous, and the 'Rest and Digest' system would efficiently get our minds and bodies back to the healthy activities of absorbing food, recovery injuries, and processing memories, experiences, and other mental problems. We didn't utilize to believe so-- however, brand-new research studies into the vagus nerve are bringing up proof to the contrary.

Working 'In reverse.'

Our muscles, food digestion, cardiovascular system, endocrine system, and so on are informed what to do by messages brought from the brain by our nerves, and they react appropriately. Numerous individuals think that this is a one-way system-- messages come from the brain, and the organs comply with.

Researchers have actually discovered something comparable to the 'center' in the vagus nerve. It's not the best example. However, it does appear that the capability to work and find with your vagus nerve is simply as efficient at 'focusing' you as taking a sedative.

Basically, the Vagus Nerve reverses the circulation of details-- rather than orders streaming from your brain to your body, the nerve is rather taking some extremely strong recommendations from the body back to the brain. It will communicate this message to the brain, which (9 times out of 10) will then reduce control over to the parasympathetic anxious system, permitting you to unwind, rest, and absorb.

When the parasympathetic nervous system has control, we can get a much deeper idea than we are when the understanding nerve system remains in control (when our instant survival is not at stake, the brain is more ready to manage time to reflect). This maybe describes why the deep breathing and physical relaxation elements of meditation assist in such exceptional consideration and self-exploration.

Mind/Body Connection

Western viewpoint has actually long battled with a significant dichotomy between the body and the mind. Given that the time of the Ancient Greek's, we have actually tended to think that the body and the mind are different entities capable just of interacting with each other, however not truly fundamentally connected. The mind has actually been held to be the body's exceptional-- something which not just manages the body; however, it can and must be utilized to reduce it in numerous cases.

This 'Mind-Body Difference' can hold itself accountable for a host of modern-day ills, not least amongst them being the concept that it does not matter what we finish with our bodies, which providing into physical desires is outrageous. To this, we can trace (in some way) weight problems, sexual pity, and an entire host of other problems.

Buddhists in basic, by contrast, understand that the body and mind belong to a meaningful whole, which affects one another and are crucial to one another's health and wellbeing. Our growing clinical understanding about the function that the vagus nerve and how synergistic body/mind actually location might permit a more holistic view of the whole human, possibly causing a much healthier, more considerate mindset towards our bodies.

Naturally, it is most likely to take a long time to alter an idea as deep-rooted as the mind-body difference. However, we can maybe utilize our understanding of the vagus nerve's operation in relation to meditation to assist those who doubt the advantages of ancient Buddhist meditation.

It must be kept in mind that any response to meditation is an extremely private thing, and the sort of deep self-knowledge promoted by extensive meditational programs might not appropriate for everybody. As we find out more, we can ideally work on methods in which to use Buddhist methods in customized methods, which can assist more of those in requirement.

GASTROPARESIS

Gastroparesis is a condition that impacts the typical spontaneous motion of the muscles (motility) in your stomach. In fact, the gastric intestinal system is regulated by strong muscular contractions. If you are gastroparesis, the motility of your abdomen is hindered or doesn't work, so that it does not clear your belly properly.

Specific medications, such as opioid painkillers, some antidepressants, and hypertension and allergic reaction medications, can cause slow stomach emptying and trigger comparable signs. For individuals who currently have gastroparesis, these medications might make their condition even worse.

Gastroparesis can interfere with regular food digestion, trigger queasiness and throwing up, and trigger issues with blood sugar levels and nutrition. There's no treatment for gastroparesis, modifications to your diet plan, along with medication, can use some relief.

SIGNS

Symptoms and signs of gastroparesis consist of:

- Throwing up
- Queasiness
- A sensation of fullness after consuming simply a couple of bites
- Throwing up undigested food consumed a couple of hours previously
- Heartburn
- Stomach bloating
- Stomach discomfort
- Modifications in blood glucose levels
- Absence of cravings
- Weight reduction and poor nutrition

Many individuals with gastroparesis do not have any visible symptoms and signs.

When to see a medical professional

If you have any indications or signs that stress you, make a visit with your medical professional.

CAUSES

It's not constantly clear what results in gastroparesis. In lots of cases, gastroparesis is thought to be triggered by damage to a nerve that manages the stomach muscles (vagus nerve).

The vagus nerve assists handle the intricate procedures in your gastrointestinal system, consisting of signifying the muscles in your stomach to an agreement and push food into the little intestinal tract. A broken vagus nerve can't send out signals usually to your abdominal muscle. This might trigger food to stay in your stomach longer, instead of move usually into your little intestinal tract to be absorbed.

The vagus nerve can be harmed by illness, such as diabetes, or by surgical treatment to the stomach or little intestinal tract.

Threat elements

Aspects that can increase your danger of gastroparesis:

- Diabetes
- Abdominal or esophageal surgical treatment
- Infection, normally an infection

- Particular medications that slow the rate of stomach emptying, such as narcotic discomfort medications
- Scleroderma (a connective tissue illness)
- Nerve system illness, such as Parkinson's illness or several sclerosis
- Hypothyroidism (low thyroid)

Females are most likely to establish gastroparesis than are guys

PROBLEMS

Gastroparesis can trigger a number of issues, such as:

- Extreme dehydration. Continuous throwing up can trigger dehydration
- Poor nutrition. Poor hunger can indicate you do not take in adequate calories, or you might be not able to soak up sufficient nutrients due to throwing up

Undigested food that stays and solidifies in your stomach. Undigested food in your stomach can solidify into a strong mass called a bezoar. If they avoid food from passing into your little intestinal tract, Bezoars can trigger queasiness and throwing up and might be deadly.

Gastroparesis does not trigger diabetes, regular modifications in the rate and quantity of food passing into the little bowel can trigger unpredictable modifications in blood sugar levels. In turn, bad control of blood sugar levels makes gastroparesis even worse.

- Reduced lifestyle. A severe flare-up of signs can make it hard to keep and work up with other duties

Medical diagnosis

Several of the following tests have confirmed the medical diagnosis of gastroparesis.

Barium x-ray

In fact, after 12 hours of fasting, the stomach is empty of all calories. Gastroparesis is most probable if the x-ray shows food in the stomach. One day a gastroparesis person can usually absorb a meal, offering an incorrectly regular test result.

Barium beefsteak meal

The amount of time it takes to digest the barium meal and leave the stomach gives the doctor an understanding of how well the stomach functions. Those with diabetes-related gastroparesis also take milk, so that the meal of barium beefsteak is beneficial.

Radioisotope gastric-emptying scan

After consuming, you will lie under a maker that discovers the radioisotope and reveals an image of the food in the stomach and how rapidly it leaves the stomach. Gastroparesis is detected if more than half of the food stays in the stomach after 2 hours.

Stomach manometry

The doctor passes a thin tube into the stomach through the throat. The conduit contains a tubing to contain liquids and solid carbohydrates, monitoring the stomach's muscular and electrical function.

Blood tests

The physician might likewise purchase lab tests to examine blood counts and to determine chemical and electrolyte levels.

To eliminate reasons for gastroparesis besides diabetes, the medical professional might do an upper endoscopy or an ultrasound.

Upper endoscopy

After giving you a sedative, the doctor passes through the mouth a long, thin tube called an endoscope and guided it carefully into the stomach through the esophagus. The medical practitioner will look at the stomach lining and check for any complications through the endoscope.

Ultrasound

To dismiss gallbladder illness or pancreatitis as a source of the issue, you might have an ultrasound test, which utilizes safe acoustic waves to specify the shape and describe of the gallbladder and pancreas.

Treatment

The main treatment objective for gastroparesis associated with diabetes is to gain back control of blood glucose levels. It is essential to keep in mind that in a lot of cases, treatment does not treat gastroparesis-- it is typically a persistent condition.

Insulin for blood sugar control

Your food is being taken in more gradually and at unforeseeable times if you have gastroparesis. To manage blood sugar, you might require it.

- Take insulin more frequently.
- Take your insulin after you consume rather than previously.
- Inspect your blood sugar levels often after you administer and consume insulin whenever needed.

Your physician will provide you particular directions based upon your specific requirements.

Medication

A number of drugs are utilized to deal with gastroparesis. Your medical professional might attempt various drugs or mixes of drugs to discover the most reliable treatment.

Metoclopramide (Reglan)

This drug promotes stomach muscle contractions to assist in empty food. It likewise assists lower queasiness and throwing up.

Erythromycin

This antibiotic likewise enhance stomach emptying. It works by increasing the contractions that move food through the stomach. Adverse effects are queasiness, throwing up, and stomach cramps.

Domperidone

The Fda is evaluating domperidone, which has actually been utilized somewhere else worldwide to deal with gastroparesis. It is a promotility representative, like metoclopramide. Domperidone likewise aids with queasiness.

Other medications

Other medications might be utilized to deal with issues and signs related to gastroparesis. If you have a bezoar, the physician might utilize an endoscope to inject the medication that will liquefy it.

Meal and Food Modifications

Altering your consuming practices can assist manage gastroparesis. Or the physician or dietitian might recommend that you attempt numerous liquid meals a day up until your blood glucose levels are steady and the gastroparesis is remedied.

Fat naturally slows food digestion-- an issue you do not require if you have gastroparesis-- and fiber is tough to absorb. Prevent these foods as the indigestible part stays too long in the stomach and can form bezoars.

Feeding Tube

A jejunostomy is especially helpful when gastroparesis avoids the nutrients and medication needed to manage blood glucose levels from reaching the bloodstream. By preventing the source of the issue-- the stomach-- and putting nutrients and medication straight into the little intestinal tract, you make sure that these items are absorbed and provided to your bloodstream rapidly. A jejunostomy tube can be momentary and is utilized just if essential when gastroparesis is serious.

Parenteral Nutrition

The medical professional puts a thin tube called a catheter in a chest vein, leaving an opening to it outside the skin. Your physician will inform you what type of liquid nutrition to utilize.

This method is an alternative to the jejunostomy tube and is generally a short-lived technique to get you through a hard spell of gastroparesis. When gastroparesis is extreme and is not assisted by other techniques, parenteral nutrition is utilized just.

New Treatments

A stomach neurostimulator has actually been established to help individuals with gastroparesis. The battery-operated gadget is surgically implanted and gives off moderate electrical pulses that assist manage queasiness and throwing up connected with gastroparesis. This choice is offered to individuals whose queasiness and throwing up do not enhance with medications.

Making use of botulinum contaminant has actually been revealed to enhance stomach emptying and the signs of gastroparesis by reducing the extended contractions of the muscle in between the stomach and the little intestinal tract (pyloric sphincter). The toxic substance is injected into the pyloric sphincter.

Hope Through Research study

NIDDK's Department of Gastrointestinal Illness and Nutrition supports scientific and standard research study into intestinal motility conditions, consisting of gastroparesis.

To list a few areas, scientists examine whether speculatory drugs can relieve or mitigate symptoms of gastroparesis, such as bloating, stomach pain, tingling, or shaking up, or reduce the amount of time the abdomen needs to clear its contents after a simple meal.

Indicate Keep in mind.

Gastroparesis might happen in individuals with type 1 diabetes or type 2 diabetes

- Gastroparesis is the outcome of damage to the vagus nerve, which manages the motion of food through the gastrointestinal system. Rather of the food moving through the gastrointestinal system generally, it is maintained in the stomach
- The vagus nerve ends up being harmed after years of bad blood sugar control, leading to gastroparesis. In turn, gastroparesis adds to bad blood sugar control
- Signs of gastroparesis consist of early fullness, queasiness, throwing up, and weight-loss.
- Tests such as ASX-rays, manometry, and scanning are used to detect gastroparesis.
- Treatments consist of modifications in when and what you consume, modifications in insulin type and timing of injections, oral medications, a jejunostomy, parenteral nutrition, stomach neurostimulators, or botulinum contaminant.

DIGESTION AND THE VAGUS NERVE

When vagus function runs out whack, food digestion runs out whack. Signs can consist of heartburn or GERD, IBD, or inflammatory bowel illness like ulcerative colitis and can avoid the body from recovery Little Intestinal tract Bacterial Overgrowth (SIBO), a regular origin of Irritable Bowel Syndrome (IBS).

The vagus nerve belongs to the system that informs the stomach to put out gastrointestinal acids and juices and to begin the motion of the gut. When we chew our food, we begin the procedure of blending the fibers in our food with the gastrointestinal acids and enzymes that start to break food down, prior to it reaches the stomach, prior to streaming into the then big and little intestinal tracts.

When the vagus nerve isn't getting or sending out the ideal signals, the circulation of food-mixed-with-acid through the gut is slowed. This implies that overcrowding, including hormones and contaminants used by the body to remove from the body, in germs, yeasts, or parasites, move slowly through the intestine.

Vagus Nerve, MMC and SIBO

The moving motor complex (MMC) in the intestines is not effective with respect to the Little Intestinal tract Bacterium Overgrowth (SIBO).

I like to think about the MMC as the caboose of a little train moving through our intestinal tracts. You consume, and the chewed up food, integrated with gastrointestinal acids and enzymes, is packed onto a vehicle on the train, to be moved through your body and out as stool. Whenever you consume, the train needs to stop and return to the top of the tracks to get the brand-new food.

Decreased vagus nerve shooting is a significant factor in MMC dysregulation. The train ought to move all the method through from Central Station, the location right after your stomach (the duodenum) through to its last stop downtown, the rectum.

This needs to be a one-way journey, and the train needs to get and leave the station to the end of the roadway every 90-120 minutes. Whenever you treat, the train needs to stop and return to get this brand-new food-passenger, slowing the motion of food through your digestion tract, which can cause bacterial overgrowth and increased contaminant concern in the body.

The MMC can likewise get hindered or puzzled by injury, tension, and other life aspects, to be gone over in-depth in additional short articles.

Low Stomach Acid

Folks with IBS, heartburn, reflux, and other gastrointestinal problems typically have low stomach acid, and this too can be a vagus nerve concern. The vagus nerve triggers the cells in the stomach to launch histamine, which assists the body to launch the stomach acid you require to break down your food.

Low B12 Levels Can Make You Feel Horrible

Lots of people with persistent gastrointestinal issues likewise have low B12 levels, which is typically due, in part, to not having enough vagus stimulation of the parietal cells in the gut, which results in low intrinsic aspects. Intrinsic aspect is the chemical that processes B12 in the stomach, and the cells that launch it can be injured and even eliminated by consuming foods we're delicate or adverse or by having without treatment heartburn, gut infections, or swelling.

The function of these cells can be slowed by improper vagus nerve stimulation-- if the gut isn't getting the "All Systems Go" signal from the brain, why would your stomach utilize all that energy to make B12?

Low B12 levels are connected to tiredness, anxiety, stress and anxiety, memory issues and dementia, nerve issues such as feeling numb or tingling, the weak point in muscles, GI signs such as irregularity, gas, diarrhea or absence of hunger.

Lions and hormonal agents

I wish to return to discussing Lions here-- both genuine and thought of.

When the vagus nerve is over or under-active, the brain's hypothalamus isn't signifying the brain's pituitary gland properly, and the downstream signal to the adrenal glands gets puzzled. This system is understood as the HPA Axis, and when this interaction is affected, a number of hormonal agents can get over- or under-produced (CRH, ACTH, and cortisol).

That is to state:

Your body can get set off into believing either that All The Lions Are Chasing You Constantly, or that there is not a single lion out there on the planet, absolutely nothing to range from, absolutely nothing to do, why trouble being present and awake to the lion-free world

This can result in a mix of tiredness, absence of inspiration, stress and anxiety, sleeping disorders, and typically, a case of the blahs. Vagus nerve stimulation contributes to assisting the body to comprehend when a scenario is a Real Lion, and when it's simply your employer being your manager or a looming due date that seems like doom.

Body clock

An extremely modern-day issue that I see daily in my clients is a change in circadian rhythm or our body's natural sleep/wake signaling. The blue light in each screen we use imitated the sun, which told our bodies it was time to be wake (while the lions were wake), and that melatonin should not be removed from our brains by our pineal glands.

I understand how appealing it is to examine social networks prior to bed, and I understand I'm not getting any fans by advising you to check out a paper book prior to bed .however, there are a couple of things your body desires more.

The vagus nerve sends signals from the circadian nerve center in the brain, and the impact of circadian dysregulation enters both instructions. Disrupting circadian circulation affects the brain, and changes in regular melatonin and another level of hormone agents prior to bed can cause vagus nerve problems, which affect your body as a whole.

The circadian control center in the brain sends out signals to your gastrointestinal system and lungs to produce mucin, the compound that keeps your essential organs well-lubricated and healthy, however just if it's getting the best signals to do so.

HOW TO COPE WITH YOUR VAGUS NERVE

In your everyday life, how often do you experience anxiety?

If you are too worried, get trapped or even experience nausea, chest pain, and heart palpitations in irrational thinking.

Through manipulating the vagus nerve, you can discover a basic but highly effective method for normal interactions with anxiety. This powerful technique can be utilized all over the place to alleviate stress and anxiety, at home, on the way and, naturally, in the terrible meetings.

Were you aware of the FDA's approval for an operating device to treat depression successfully by regularly stimulating the vagus nerve?

I hope you won't need surgery, however. Through following certain basic breathing techniques, you will benefit from mildly activated nerves.

What's the vagus nerve, then?

The vagus nervous system is the most important part of the sympathetic system of the nervous system, which calms you by controlling your relaxation response.

It emerges in the abdomen as the brain and "travers" spread tongue fibers (like acetylcholine, prolactin, vasopressine, oxytocin), monitor digestion, metallicity and, of course, soothe the answer), spreading language fibers, the pharynx, the vocal chord, the lungs, back, intestines and drums. It can be used to prevent digestion or otherwise.

Vagus nerve is used as a link between the mind and the body, and cables are the back of emotions and intestinal impulses. The key to monitoring your mind and anxiety is to trigger the soothing nervous pathways of your parasympathetic system.

This part of the nervous system can not be controlled, but the vagus nerve can be stimulated indirectly:

Immerse your face in cold water (scuba reflex)

Tentative of exhaling from a blocked airway (Valsalva maneuver).

You can do this while you breathe out by keeping your mouth closed and pinching your nose. The vagus nerve and vagus activate significantly increased pressure within the cavity.

Singing

Naturally, the reinforcement of this living nervous system will have a great advantage, and the best way to do it is by practicing your breathing.

Breathe your diaphragm

This definition now has to be incorporated. You have to breathe your diaphragm the first thing. This is the foundation of healthy breathing and anxiety.

Your breathing muscle is the diaphragm. It is belled, and it is shaped (or should flatten) when inhaled, it acts as a tube in the thoracic cavity that produces a pressure that spreads the lungs, pulling them out with oxygen.

On the other hand, it sets the viscera down and out, stretches the abdomen. It creates pressure. Good breathing is therefore defined as breathing in the abdomen or abdomen.

Breathe partially closed with the glottis

Glottis is behind your tongue, and it is covered while you hold your breath. Here we want it to be locked partly. You get the impression as you exhale and make a sound of "Hhhhh" to rinse your glasses, but not making the sound.

It's the way you relax as you sleep, and you're going to rummage a little.

You are: by controlling the glottis

Inhalation and exhalation airflow control Stimulate your vagus nerve.

Now is the time to apply this principle through this 7-11 diaphragmatic breathing technique.

- Dip into your nose with your glottis partially shut, like making a sound of "Hhhhh" for a number of 7.
- Hold for a moment, your breath.

- Exhale your nose (or mouth) with your glottis partially closed, just like making a "Hhhh" sound like an eleventh count.
- This is a breath cycle; it takes 6-12 cycles to monitor the results

CONCLUSION

Simply put, the vagus nerve is the master and control of your major organs in your inner nerve center. This is the longest ever cranial in the brain that starts behind the ears and attaches to every major body organ. This transfer fiber from your brain system to all your visceral organs and is essentially the head of your inner nervous center. The term vagus literally means "hiker" because it travels across their entire body from the brain to the reproductive organs and touches everything. In relation to the relation of the mind-body, the vagus nerve is important since it enters all major organs except the surreal and thyroid drums.

For each organ with which it is in contact, this is an essential nerve. It helps manage the anxiety and depression in the brain. We interact tightly with the vaguely connected nerve, which allows our speech to communicate and regulates eye contact and movements. This nerve can also affect the right release of hormones in the body that sustain our physical and mental processes stable.

The vagus nerve increases the acidity and digestive juice production of the intestine to promote food absorption. It can also be beneficial when activated to absorb vitamin B12. And you can expect serious intestinal problems such as colitis, IBS, so Re-flux, to name a few when they do not work properly. Reflux symptoms can be caused by a vagus nerve injury because it affects the esophagus as well. It is the undesirable expression of the esophagus that causes conditions like Gerd and Reflux.

The nerve is also used to control heart rate and blood pressure to prevent heart disease. While blood glycolysis is controlled in your liver and pancreas, diabetes is prevented by this nerve. Once the bile is passed, the vagus nerve helps release the bile, which removes toxins and breaks down fat. In the bladder, this nerve stimulates the general operation of the liver, increases blood flow and enhances the corporal filtration. When the vagus nerve enters the spleen, it reduces inflammation throughout the target organs. This nerve even has the power to control female orgasms and fertility. An ineffective or blocked vagus nerve may cause disturbances across the body and spirit.

You can easily conclude that any mental, body, or spiritual disorder, disease or ill health can be reversed or even cured by stimulating and stimulating your vagus nerve if you know that it is associated with the major organs and functions properly. Therefore, the good effects on such things as anxiety, heart disease, headaches and migraines, fibromyalgia, alcohol addiction, respiration, intestinal problems, memories, mood issues, MS and cancer are seen really from vagus nerves stimulation.

The vagus nerve is activated several times, such as music or talking, smiling, yoga, sleep, breathing exercises and just looking to name a few. The muscles in the back of your throat are relaxed by music and laughter. Modern fitness and general exercise improve intestinal fluids that activate the vagus. Regimented yoga can also enhance movement nerve stimulation, but meditation and OM can boost vagus nerve stimulation. There is one thing in common in all these ways to stimulate the vagus nerve: vibration!!

Resonant organ level observations are made throughout the world by doctors to help the body recover its health through the transfusion of illnesses and conditions like anxiety, PTSD, migraines, insomnia, memory problems, chronic pain, sleep disturbances, and cancer. Dr. Gaynor, Oncology Director at the Center for Cancer Prevention Strang-Cornell in New York and author of Sounds of Healing, says, "You really can look at cancer as a form of disharmony." We know that sound and music have profound effects on the immune system, which clearly are very much related to cancer. "The study also included Alzheimer's disease in April 2016. Researchers at the University of Toronto, the University of Wilfrid Laurier, and Baycrest Center Hospitals conducted a study in the various stages of the disease, which was subject to 40 hertz sound simulation. They acknowledged with intellect, comprehension and alertness" promising "outcomes. One of the authors of the results, Lee Bartel, said," Pieces of the brain is at the same frequency, and that frequency is approximately 40 Hz. And if you become older, if it is too little, then you can't get a short-term memory for a long time, two brain pieces, like the Thalamus and the Hippocampus that you want to speak to each other. Tomatis said he had handled a wide range of conditions effectively through the sound because they had all been related to issues with the inner ear. Only a handful of the issues he successfully dealt with include stuttering, depression, ADD, problems with concentration and balance.

Another study shows that ADD helps children through the Tomatis approach. "The results show significant improvements in the processing speed, phonological comprehension, phonemic decoding efficiency in hearing, conduct and audition behavior in the Tomatis community as opposed to the non-Tomatis Community."

Do Not Go Yet; One Last Thing To Do
I would be very happy if you would give a short
review of Amazon if you liked the book or found it
useful. Your encouragement really makes a difference,
and I personally read all reviews to get your input and
develop the book.

Thanks for your assistance again!